A commonsense approach to coronary care
A PROGRAM

A commonsense approach to coronary care

A PROGRAM

MARIELLE ORTIZ VINSANT, R.N., B.S.

Instructor, Department of Nursing Research and Development,
Jackson Memorial Hospital, Miami, Florida

MARTHA I. SPENCE, R.N., B.S., M.N.

Part-time Instructor, Department of Nursing Research
and Development, Jackson Memorial Hospital,
Miami, Florida

DIANNE CHAPELL HAGEN, R.N., B.S.

Instructor, Orange County Community College,
School of Nursing, Middletown, New York

SECOND EDITION

with 439 *illustrations; original drawings by* Marcellino Obaya

The C. V. Mosby Company

Saint Louis 1975

VH/VH/B   9   8   7   6   5   4

To

LOUIS LEMBERG, M.D.

AGUSTIN CASTELLANOS, Jr., M.D.

AZUCENA G. ARCEBAL, M.D.

GLORIA STEFFENS, R.N., M.S.

who gave us the autonomy and inspiration to grow

Foreword

This book is a good example of a premise that arose twenty-two centuries ago, namely, that teaching is an art rather than a science. Unfortunately this principle is often neglected in our technified age. To achieve their purpose the authors of this book have addressed human beings as individuals, not anonymous persons. Readers must be well aware of these aims if they are to obtain full benefit from the material presented. They must also recognize that it is dangerous and antididactic to apply the goals and methods of science to all aspects of learning. Gilbert Highet has repeatedly emphasized that a strictly scientific relationship (either verbal or written) between teacher and pupil is inadequate and undesirable. Naturally, some coherence is required in all presentations, but this does not remove the emotional ingredients.

The "system" used in this book arose after hundreds of live encounters in the form of spontaneous (or conventional) lectures, dialogues, and discussions. Hence, it was based on a person-to-person relation in which readers must act as inquisitive pupils—true interlocutors who can find themselves believing or doubting, yet persistently *thinking*, about the various approaches to coronary care which they would not have looked upon in exactly the same fashion. Unless readers work themselves into the proper mental framework, it is possible that this approach might appear too complex, highly dogmatic; or, for some, extraordinarily simple. But in any case, the stimulation created in the minds of readers is even more important than the factual information. Whereas not all scientific statements can be proven, the desire to learn can be experienced by all.

Agustin Castellanos, Jr., M.D.

Preface

We first became aware of the need for a new approach to coronary care training while teaching nurses in a course sponsored by The Florida Regional Medical Program and the Florida Heart Association.

Initially we used a traditional fragmented approach, but this methodology met with only moderate success. As we were stimulated to question and learn more concerning clinical cardiology, we became more disillusioned with this approach. It did not provide the nurse with a basis for realistically and systematically solving patient problems. Subsequently, we developed our own methods for simplification, organization, and practical presentation of subject matter. As this approach met with success, we wondered if others might also find it meaningful.

Our approach is based on a thorough knowledge of normal anatomy and physiology. Utilizing knowledge of anatomy and physiology, the student is able to deduce the clinical consequences of pathological changes. For example, knowledge of the anatomy of the coronary artery system enables the practitioner to anticipate the types of complications that will be associated with coronary artery occlusion.

In this book we do not attempt to deal with all aspects of coronary artery disease. We will focus on the major problems associated with acute myocardial infarction. We do not emphasize psychological and rehabilitative aspects of coronary care because they do not lend themselves to our programming format, and there is other excellent current literature available by experts in this field. It is definitely not our intention to minimize the obvious importance of these concepts in the area of coronary care.

It was our aim to simulate as closely as possible our classroom situation. We believe that the students' interest increases as they are encouraged to participate. By participating, students are also given a means of evaluating their understanding and learning of the topics discussed. We chose the programmed format for this book because we felt that it would be the best to fulfill these aims. Information is presented in a comprehensive, correlated form. We believe that memorization is a crutch, not an effective learning tool. Therefore, readers are encouraged to use their reasoning powers to a maximum and keep memorization to a minimum.

This book is directed toward beginner and advanced practitioner alike. No previous knowledge of cardiology is necessary, though we feel that those who have some experience will also find it useful. Units 1, 2, and 3 have been revised to make them more meaningful for the beginning student. Other additions, such as the hemodynamic information in Unit 7, have been made to increase the text's relevance for the more advanced practitioner. More complete pharmacological information is provided in Unit 8.

This text is so constructed that each unit is built upon the preceding unit. The student is cautioned *not* to read isolated segments of the book. Cross references, reviews, and repetition are provided to maintain the continuity of the units. Readers who do not understand the answer given should refer to the previous unit discussing that topic.

We would like to acknowledge and thank Dr. Agustin "Tino" Castellanos, our teacher, philosopher, and friend, for his patience and encouragement, for always being available when we needed him, and for never complaining while proofing this text; Dr. Louis Lemberg, for his willingness to sponsor us in all our endeavors, for his dedication and commitment to coronary care nurse training, and for keeping us clinically oriented; Dr. Azucena Arcebal, for her unique ability to present complex material in a simplified but accurate fashion, for her willingness to always share her knowledge with us, and for treating us as peers; and The Florida Regional Medical Program and the Florida Heart Association, for giving us the opportunity to become involved in coronary care nurse training.

We would also like to acknowledge others who have taught us during the past five years: Gloria Steffens, R.N., Dr. Joan Mayer, Dr. Robert Boucek, Dr. Ramanuja Iyengar, Dr. Ronald Fox, Dr. Charles Roeth, Shirley Mason, R.N., Judy Mercure, R.N., Dr. Jeffrey Raskin, Dr. John Hildreth, Dr. Alvaro Martinez, Barouh Berkovits, Enoch Sprague, Dr. Earl Barron, Dr. Sayfie, Bruce Raykowski, Dr. Mary Richards, Dr. James Barkin, Dr. Ali Gharamani, Dr. Hooshang Balooki, Dr. Abellardo Vargas, Dr. Sung, Dr. Dan Clark, and Dr. Joseph Civetta.

For their time spent in proofing and production of this text, we would like to acknowledge Dr. Robert Zoble, Dr. Salvatore DiGiorgi, Dr. Francis Worthington, Dr. Michael Gordon, LaVonne Hendrix, R.N., Theresa Nuzum, R.N., and Annie Neasman, R.N.

We also thank our illustrator, Marcellino Obaya, and our secretaries, Charlotte Griggs, Claudine Collier, Chris Michaud, and Ann Trager. We would like to extend a special thank you to Laura Bott, who not only was one of our original secretaries but also completely typed this first revision.

For their encouragement and overall assistance, we acknowledge our parents, Dr. and Mrs. Arturo C. Ortiz, Mr. and Mrs. Harold Inglis, Mrs. J. M. Chapell, and Mr. Hank Spence.

Marielle Ortiz Vinsant
Martha I. Spence
Dianne Chapell Hagen

Contents

A commonsense approach to coronary care
A PROGRAM

Anatomy and physiology

1 The primary function of the heart is *mechanical*. It serves as a pump to deliver oxygenated blood to the body tissues in an attempt to meet their metabolic demands.
The amount of blood put out by the heart per minute is known as the *cardiac output* (CO).

2 Cardiac output is a product of *ventricular rate* × *stroke volume* (CO = VR × SV).
Variations in cardiac output can thus be produced by altering the

_____ _____ or the _____ _____.   *ventricular rate;*
                                                      stroke volume

3 The *heart rate* is primarily determined by the integrity of the heart's electrical system and the influence of the autonomic nervous system.
The *stroke volume* is primarily determined by the pumping efficiency of the cardiac muscle and the blood volume returning to the heart.

4 *Let us review:* In an attempt to meet the demands of the tissues, the heart pumps out a certain amount of oxygenated blood per minute. This amount of blood is known as the _____ _____.   *cardiac output*

Cardiac output is a product of _____ _____ and   *ventricular rate*

_____ _____.   *stroke volume*

5 Normally, the body compensates for rises and falls in stroke volume and heart rate so that as one increases the other decreases. Therefore, when the trained athlete increases his cardiac muscle mass and thus his stroke volume, the heart rate *(increases/decreases)*.   *decreases*

6 If the body cannot compensate for a fall in heart rate by increasing the stroke volume or, conversely, for a fall in stroke volume by increasing the rate, the cardiac output then *(rises/falls)*.   *falls*

7 If the demands of the tissues for oxygen are not met because of this fall in cardiac output, the patient may begin to exhibit symptoms such as:
1. Dizziness, fainting, or mental confusion
2. Cold clammy skin
3. Decreased urinary output

8 When *symptoms* develop because of a fall in heart rate, it is said

that the patient is experiencing a _____ fall in cardiac   *symptomatic*
output. The heart rate is too slow for this particular patient regardless of the exact number of beats per minute.

9 When the heart muscle has been damaged or injured as in acute myocardial infarction (MI) resulting in heart failure, the stroke

1

volume *(increases/decreases)*. The body compensates to maintain   *decreases*

cardiac output by increasing the _____ _____.   *heart rate*
One of the earliest signs of heart failure is *(fast/slow)* rates.   *fast*

MECHANICAL STRUCTURES

10   The heart is divided into a right and left side by a muscular structure known as the *septum*.

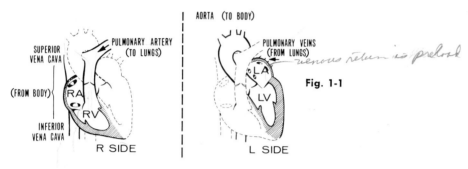

Fig. 1-1

11   The right and left sides of the heart *differ* in: (1) function; (2) musculature; (3) valvular structure.

12   The function of the right side of the heart is to deliver *unoxygen-*

ated blood from the _____ to the _____.   *body*   *lungs*
The function of the left side of the heart is to deliver *oxygenated*

blood from the _____ to the _____.   *lungs*   *body*

13   Blood enters the right side of the heart via *veins*, the superior vena

cava and the _____ _____ _____.   *inferior vena cava*
Blood leaves the right side of the heart via an *artery*, the

_____ _____.   *pulmonary artery*

Blood enters the left side of the heart via four *veins*, the

_____ _____.   *pulmonary veins*

Blood leaves the left side of the heart via an *artery*, the _____.   *aorta*
Note: Veins carry blood toward the heart.
        Arteries carry blood away from the heart.

14   The right side of the heart has *thinner musculature*, since it projects its volume against minimal resistance in the pulmonary circulation.
The left side of the heart has *thicker musculature* since it projects its volume against *(greater/lesser)* resistance in the peripheral circulation.   *greater*

15   Each side of the heart has two sets of valves. Valves serve as separators and further divide each side of the heart into a receiving chamber, the *atrium*, and an ejecting chamber, the *ventricle*. Atrio-

ventricular (A-V) valves separate the atria from the _____.   *ventricles*
Semilunar valves separate the ventricles from the vessels leaving them.

16   The A-V valve in the right side of the heart is the *tricuspid* valve.

2

It separates the right atrium from the _____ _____.   *right ventricle*

The *A-V* valve in the left side of the heart is the mitral valve. It

separates the left atrium from the _____ _____. The A-V   *left ventricle*
valves on both sides of the heart are supported by rope-like structures known as *chordae tendineae*, which attach to papillary mus-

cles. The _____ muscles allow for normal movement of the   *papillary*

_____ valves.   *A-V*

17 The *semilunar* valve in the right side of the heart is the *pulmonary*
valve. It separates the right ventricle from the vessel leaving it,

the _____ _____.   *pulmonary artery*
The semilunar valve in the left side of the heart is the *aortic* valve.

It separates the left ventricle from its outflow vessel, the _____.   *aorta*

18 IN SUMMARY:

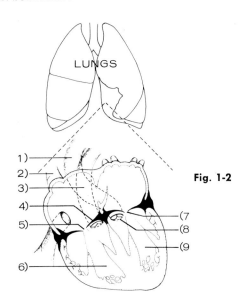

Fig. 1-2

Key

1 Aorta
2 Superior vena cava
3 Pulmonary artery
4 Pulmonary valve
5 Tricuspid valve
6 Right ventricle
7 Mitral valve
8 Aortic valve
9 Left ventricle

Table 1

		Right ventricle	*Left ventricle*
Function	1.	Delivers *unoxygenated* blood *from body to lungs*	1. Delivers *oxygenated* blood *from lungs to body*
	2.	Projects its volume against minimal resistance—*the lungs*	2. Projects its volume against maximum resistance—*the body*
Musculature	3.	Thin walls	3. Thick walls
Valves	4.	*A-V valve:* tricuspid	4. *A-V valve:* mitral
	5.	*Semilunar valve:* pulmonary	5. *Semilunar valve:* aortic

Since more of the work of the heart is performed by the *(right/*
left) ventricle, the major cardiac problems may be traced to the   *left*
(right/left) ventricle.   *left*

Myocardial infarction occurs almost exclusively in the *(right/left)*   *left*
ventricle.

The major valves affected in cardiac disease are the _____ and   *mitral*

_____ valves, located on the *(right/left)* side of the heart.   *aortic*   *left*

MECHANICAL ACTIVITY

19 The mechanical activity of the heart consists of a period of contraction known as *systole* and a period of relaxation and filling
known as *diastole*.

Atrial contraction may also be called atrial _____. Ventricular   *systole*

contraction may also be called ventricular _____.   *systole*
Note: Ventricular systole corresponds to the apical pulse.

20 The right and left atria fill and contract together. For our purposes,
then, they may be considered as a single functional unit. The right
and left ventricles fill and contract together. They may also be considered as a single functional unit.

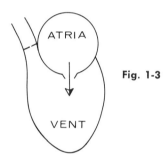

Fig. 1-3

21 The heart sounds serve as parameters for clinically recognizing
the mechanical events of the heart.
Heart sounds are essentially produced by closure of the valves, although the exact mechanics involved in production of the sound
are more complex (see Unit 7).

22 During ventricular systole, the valves between the atria and the
ventricles must close so that blood may be ejected into the blood
vessels. Since ventricular systole is considered to be the first mechanical event, the sound produced by closure of these valves is

known as the first heart sound, or _____. S_1
The "lub" heard with a stethoscope is also representative of this

event. S_1 is produced by closure of the _____ valves and marks   *A-V*
the onset of ventricular *(systole/diastole)*.   *systole*

23 During ventricular diastole the semilunar valves are closed so that
blood only enters the ventricles from the atria.
Remember: The semilunar valves separate the ventricles from the

_____ leaving them. Since diastole is the second event of the   *vessel*
cardiac cycle, the sound produced by closure of these valves is

known as _____. S_2
The "dub" heard with a stethoscope is also representative of this
event.

4

S$_2$ is produced by closure of the _____ valves and marks the onset of ventricular *(systole/diastole)*.

semilunar

diastole

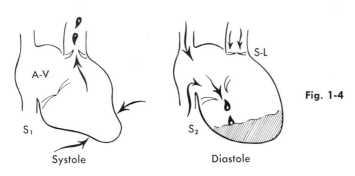

Fig. 1-4

Systole   Diastole

24 It is important to note that closure of the A-V valves occurs not only as a result of ventricular contraction but also as a result of pressure changes in the *ventricular chamber*.

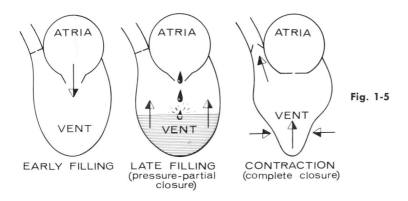

Fig. 1-5

EARLY FILLING   LATE FILLING   CONTRACTION
                  (pressure-partial   (complete closure)
                  closure)

Pressure increases in the ventricular chambers as they fill. As a result of this pressure the valves begin to close passively. When the ventricles contract, this mechanical event actively completes closure of the valves.

Closure of the A-V valves, then, is a result of both _____ and

_____ mechanical activity.

active

passive

25 Atrial events also play a role during ventricular systole and diastole. Atrial systole occurs during ventricular diastole. It contributes the last boost of blood into the ventricles before ventricular systole.

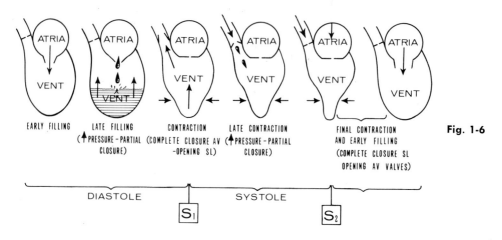

EARLY FILLING   LATE FILLING   CONTRACTION   LATE CONTRACTION   FINAL CONTRACTION   Fig. 1-6

(↑PRESSURE–PARTIAL   (COMPLETE CLOSURE AV   (↑PRESSURE–PARTIAL   AND EARLY FILLING

CLOSURE)   –OPENING SL)   CLOSURE)   (COMPLETE CLOSURE SL

OPENING AV VALVES)

DIASTOLE   SYSTOLE

S_1 S_2

Systole (ventricular) occurs between S_1 and S_2.

Diastole (ventricular) occurs between S_2 and S_1.

ELECTRICAL ACTIVITY OF THE HEART

27 The heart has an intrinsic electrical system that allows for the origination and transmission of an electrical impulse.
The *electrical activity* of the heart consists of: (1) the *electrical
stimulus* (the initiating factor); (2) *depolarization* (the prolifer-
ating factor).

28 Essentially this electrical activity *prepares* the heart to contract.

The heart is prepared to contract by _____ activity.   *electrical*

29 The electrical activity of the heart may be recorded on paper. This
record is known as the electrocardiogram, or *ECG*.
Evidence of electrical activity, then, is manifested on the _____.   *ECG*

Relationship to mechanical activity

30 Electrical activity *precedes* mechanical activity.
The *mechanical activity* consists of *contraction*. The heart can then
function as a *pump*.

31 The mechanical activity of the heart is noted by the presence of

_____. Myocardial contraction results in the formation of   *contraction*
a *pulse*.
Evidence of mechanical activity, then, is manifested by the _____.   *pulse*

32 Mechanical activity is the most important because it is the assur-

ance of actual _____ action.   *pump*
When there is electrical activity there is *usually* mechanical activity. However, electrical activity may occur *without* mechanical activity.
For every beat on the ECG there is usually a corresponding

_____. However, there can be beats on the ECG *without* a corre-   *pulse*

sponding _____. Clinically, then, the best evidence of mechanical   *pulse*

activity is the _____.   *pulse*

Properties of cardiac cells

33 The heart cells have four main properties, which allow for the integration of electrical and mechanical activity.
1. *automaticity*—the ability to *initiate* an impulse or stimulus
2. *excitability*—the ability to *respond* to an impulse or stimulus
3. *conductivity*—the ability to *transmit* impulses to other areas
4. *contractility*—the ability to respond to this electrical impulse with *pump* action

34 The heart can initiate its own impulse (_____), respond   *automaticity*

to this impulse (_____), and transmit this impulse   *excitability*

(_____). These are *(electrical/mechanical)* properties.   *conductivity; electrical*

35 *Contractility* is the _____ property of the heart.   *mechanical*

The electrical conduction system

36 The conduction pathway normally begins in the *sinoatrial* (S-A) *node*. The electrical stimulus is normally initiated in this area. Thus

the _____ node is called the pacemaker of the   *sinoatrial (S-A)*
heart.

The S-A node

37 The S-A node is located in the right atrium close to the superior vena cava. It is a specialized piece of tissue that can periodically initiate its own impulses. The S-A node, therefore, is said to have

the property of _____.   *automaticity*

38 Normally, the S-A node initiates its own impulses at a rate of 60 to 100 per minute.
Note: Other areas of the heart, such as the A-V junctional tissue, lower portions of the atria, and the His-Purkinje system in the ventricles, also have the property of automaticity. The S-A node is the normal pacemaker. It initiates impulses at a *(faster/slower)* rate   *faster*

than the other areas of the heart and therefore sets the _____ of   *pace*
the heart.

39 The S-A node is innervated by the autonomic nervous system. Sympathetic stimulation can accelerate the S-A node to a rate up to 150 *(sinus tachycardia)*. Parasympathetic stimulation can *slow* the heart rate to less than 60 *(sinus bradycardia)*.
However, if the heart were separated from the body's nervous system, the S-A node *(could/could not)* still initiate its own impulses.   *could*

40 Once an electrical impulse is originated, it spreads throughout the conduction system and the heart muscle. This is accomplished by a process known as *depolarization*.
The pathway receiving the electrical stimulus is negatively charged *(polarized)*. It must be made positive so that the impulse may be conducted.
The process by which these changes occur is known as

_____.   *depolarization*

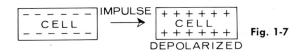
Fig. 1-7

Depolarization, then, may be considered as advancing *(positive/ negative)* charges.

           positive

41 When the impulse is released from the S-A node, it travels through the specialized conduction tissue in the atria and causes them to contract.

Note: These specialized atrial conduction fibers, which lie between the S-A node and the A-V node, are known as the internodal tracts.

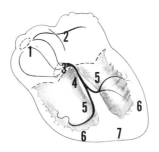

Fig. 1-8

42 The normal sequence of activation in the heart is:

1. _____   *S-A node*

2. _____   *atria*

3. _____   *A-V node*

4. _____   *bundle of His*

5. _____   *bundle branches*

6. _____   *Purkinje fibers*

7. _____   *ventricular mus-culature*

A-V junctional tissue

43 The A-V node is located in the right atrium close to the septal leaflet of the tricuspid valve.

The A-V node and the conduction tissue surrounding it are known

as the A-V _____ tissue.   *junctional*
A-V junctional tissue, like the S-A node, has the property of

_____.   *automaticity*

44 Under normal conditions an impulse from the S-A node will be released before the A-V junctional tissue can be spontaneously depolarized. The S-A node therefore normally *dominates* the A-V junc-

tional tissue and sets the _____ for the heart.   *pace*
If the S-A node is unable to maintain its normal pace, the _____   *A-V*

_____ tissue can assume control as the dominant   *junctional*

_____ of the heart.   *pacemaker*

45 Under normal conditions, the A-V junctional tissue *(is/is not)* the   *is not*
pacemaker of the heart. It initiates impulses at a rate *(faster/*

slower) than the _____ node.   *slower*   *S-A*

8

If the S-A node is injured or depressed, the _____ _____   *A-V junctional*
tissue can take over.

The rate of impulse formation in the A-V junctional tissue is normally *40 to 70* per minute.

The rate of impulse discharge in the S-A node is normally _____   *60*

_____ _____ per minute.   *to 100*

When the A-V junctional tissue assumes the role of pacemaker of
the heart, the heart rate will usually be *(faster/slower)* than when   *slower*

the heart is under the control of the _____ node.   *S-A*

46 The heart's electrical impulse delays briefly at the _____ junc-   *A-V*
tional tissue. This delay allows for atrial contraction to precede ventricular contraction. The atria are thus able to provide the last
boost of blood into the ventricles *before* ventricular contraction occurs.

This *atrial component* contributes 20 to 30% of the cardiac output.
In people with normal conduction, the atria contract *(before/after)*   *before*
the ventricles and *(add to/subtract from)* cardiac output.   *add to*

The His-Purkinje network (the ventricular conduction tissue)

47 The conduction structures in the *ventricles* consist of the *His-Purkinje network.*

Ventricular conduction tissue, therefore, may be referred to as the

_____ network.   *His-Purkinje*

48 The ventricular conduction tissue, like the A-V junctional tissue

and the S-A node, has the property of _____.   *automaticity*

Under normal conditions, an impulse from the _____ node will   *S-A*
occur before the ventricular or A-V tissue is able to spontaneously
depolarize.

The S-A node, therefore, normally *dominates both* the A-V junc-

tional and _____ tissue and functions as the   *ventricular*

_____ of the heart.   *pacemaker*

49 If *both* the S-A node and the A-V junctional tissue are unable to

maintain control of the rhythm, the _____ can assume   *ventricles*

control as the dominant _____ of the heart.   *pacemaker*
Under normal conditions, then, the ventricles *(are/are not)* the   *are not*
pacemakers of the heart.

Remember: The ventricles initiate impulses at a rate *(faster/*

slower) than either the _____ _____ or the   *slower   S-A node*

_____ _____ _____.   *A-V junctional tissue*

If both the S-A node and the A-V junctional tissue are injured or

depressed, the _____ conduction tissue can take over.   *ventricular*

50 *Let us review:* The normal pacemaker of the heart is the _____   *S-A*

_____.   *node*

If the S-A node is injured or depressed, the _____   *A-V*

_____ _____ can assume control as pacemaker   *junctional tissue*
of the heart.

9

51 The S-A node, A-V junctional tissue, and ventricular conduction tissue can all independently pace the heart because they all have the property of _____.   *automaticity*
The lower the pacemaker site in the heart, the *(faster/slower)* the   *slower*
heart rate.

THE PLANES OF THE HEART

52 Both the mechanical and electrical activity of the heart are often considered in relationship to views of the heart in different planes. Let us now consider each plane in which we view the heart.

53 A plane is a flat two-dimensional surface.
The heart may be considered as having the following dimensions:
1. width—bordered by right and left
2. height—bordered superiorly and inferiorly
3. depth—bordered anteriorly and posteriorly

Two dimensions form a _____.   *plane*

54 When a patient is viewed from the front, the dimensions observed are: (1) width, bordered by right and left; (2) height, bordered superiorly and inferiorly.

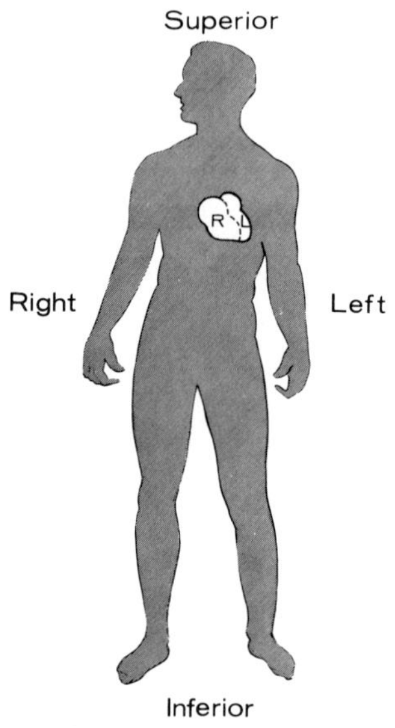

Superior

R L

Right   Left

Fig. 1-9

Inferior
FRONTAL PLANE

A two-dimensional surface is known as a _____.   *plane*

The dimensions of the frontal plane are: (1) _____, (2)   *width*

_____.   *height*

55 *Remember:* Width is bordered by _____ and _____; height is   *right   left*

bordered _____ and _____.   *superiorly   inferiorly*
Therefore, four borders serve to outline a plane. The borders of the

frontal plane are: (1) _____, (2) _____, (3) _____,   *left; right; superior*

(4) _____.   *inferior*

56 When a patient is viewed from the side in the sagittal plane the di-

mensions observed are _____ and _____.

The borders of this plane are: (1) _____, (2) _____,

(3)_____, (4) _____.

height   *depth*

superior   *inferior*

anterior   *posterior*

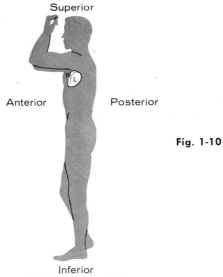

Fig. 1-10

SAGITTAL PLANE

Note: The left sagittal plane is obtained by viewing the patient from his left side.

57 When a patient is viewed horizontally, i.e., in the horizontal plane,

the dimensions observed are: (1) _____, (2) _____.

The borders of the horizontal plane are: (1) _____, (2) _____,

(3) _____, (4) _____.

width   *depth*

left   *right*

anterior   *posterior*

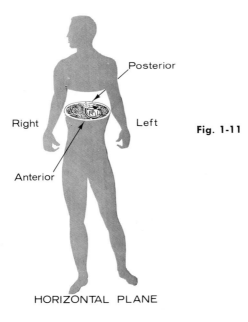

Fig. 1-11

HORIZONTAL PLANE

11

The inferior surface of the heart *(does/does not)* border the hori-   *does not*
zontal plane.

58 IN SUMMARY:

The heart may be visualized in three planes. The borders of the

frontal plane are: (1) _____, (2) _____, (3) _____,   *left; right; superior*

(4) _____.   *inferior*

The borders of the *sagittal plane* are: (1) _____, (2) _____,   *superior*   *inferior*

(3) _____, (4) _____.   *anterior*   *posterior*

The borders of the *horizontal plane* are: (1) _____, (2) _____,   *left*   *right*

(3) _____, (4) _____.   *anterior*   *posterior*

POSITION OF THE HEART WITHIN THE CHEST

59 The heart is *rotated* and positioned on its side within the chest cavity. The right ventricle lies anteriorly and the left ventricle lies posteriorly.

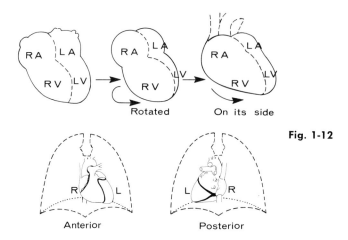

Fig. 1-12

60 Let us now isolate the left ventricle within the chest cavity:

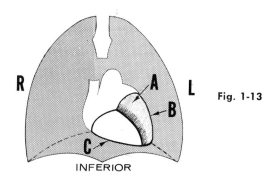

Fig. 1-13

This illustration was obtained in the _____ plane.   *frontal*

61 In Fig. 1-13, the borders visualized are: (1) _____ to _____;   *right*   *left*

(2) _____ to _____.   *superior*   *inferior*

62 In Fig. 1-13:
   A represents the *anterior* portion of the left ventricle
   B represents the *lateral* portion of the left ventricle.
   C represents the *inferior* surface of the left ventricle
   Note: The *inferior* surface of the left ventricle lies on the dia-

   phragm. Therefore it may also be called the _____   *diaphragmatic*
   surface of the heart.

63 An injury affecting area **A** of the left ventricle, then, would be

   called an _____ wall injury.   *anterior*
   An injury affecting area **C** of the left ventricle would be called an

   _____ wall injury.   *inferior*

64 The inferior surface of the heart may be better visualized in the
   sagittal plane:

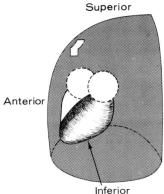

Fig. 1-14

THE CORONARY ARTERY SYSTEM

65 Like other organs in the body, the heart has its own rich blood
   supply.
   The heart receives blood for its own maintenance from two *coronary arteries*, the right and the left.

66 The coronary arteries are the first branches off the aorta. They originate from the cusps of the aortic valves in the *sinuses of Valsalva*.
   The site of origin of the coronary arteries is the sinuses of

   _____ in the _____ cusps.   *Valsalva   aortic*

67 The heart's blood supply provides blood for both its *electrical* and
   mechanical structures.
   The *electrical* structure of the heart is the *conduction system*.
   The *mechanical* structure of the heart includes the heart muscle, or
   myocardium.
   The heart's blood supply therefore provides blood to both the

   _____ structures and the _____.   *conduction;*
                                                              myocardium

The right coronary artery

68 Let us trace the pathway of each coronary artery and list the structures that each supplies:

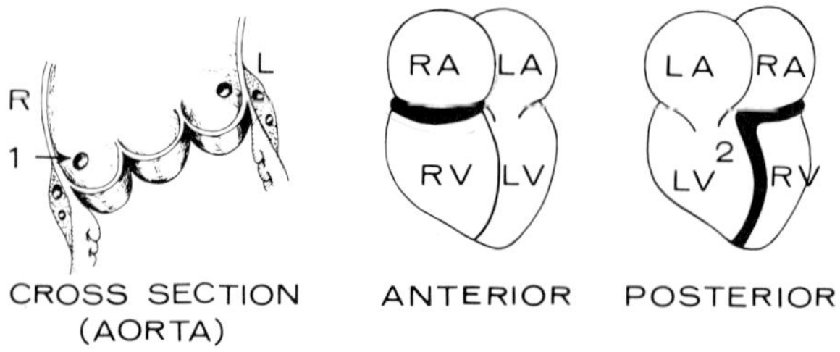

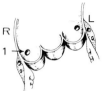
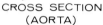
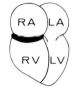

CROSS SECTION
(AORTA)   ANTERIOR   POSTERIOR

Fig. 1-15

The *right coronary artery* branches off from the _____ sinus
of Valsalva. It then proceeds to the anterior surface of the heart
and winds around to the right in the groove between the right
atrium and the right ventricle.
Note: Before reaching the surface of the heart, a branch is emitted
that supplies an important structure, the *S-A node.*

right

69 The right coronary artery then winds around the back of the heart
dividing the right atrium and the right ventricle *(anteriorly/poste-
riorly).* An important branch is given off at this point, which descends posteriorly in the groove separating the right and left ventricles. The name of this branch is the *posterior descending branch.*
Note: The right coronary artery gives a branch to the A-V node at
about the same level as the origin of the posterior descending
branch.

posteriorly

The right coronary artery, then, supplies both the _____ and the

_____ nodes.

S-A

A-V

70 As the right coronary artery winds around the back of the heart

and descends, it emits a major branch known as the _____

_____ _____.

The posterior descending also emits branches that perforate the
septum posteriorly. These are called the *septal* branches. These
branches supply a portion of the *bundle of His,* the *posterior one-
third* of the septum, and a portion of the *inferoposterior division of
the left bundle branch.*
Note: The bundle branches divide into right and _____. The left
further divides into two divisions, the posterior-inferior and the
anterior-superior.

posterior

descending branch

left

71 The right coronary artery also supplies heart _____.
The right coronary artery travels toward the *(right/left)* side of

the heart dividing the _____ _____ from the _____

_____.

The blood supply of the *right* _____ and *right* _____ is

therefore provided by the _____ coronary artery.

muscle
right

*right atrium; right
   ventricle*

atrium   ventricle

right

72 The right coronary artery also supplies a portion of the *left ventricular muscle.*
The right coronary artery emits a posterior descending branch that

separates the _____ ventricle from the left ventricle *(anteri-
orly/posteriorly).*
The right coronary artery therefore supplies a portion of the left
ventricle *posteriorly.*

right
posteriorly

73 Let us consider the left ventricle as it lies in the chest cavity:

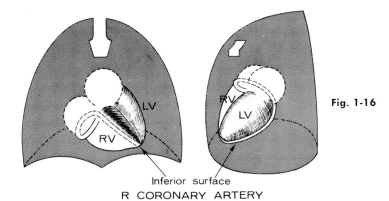

Fig. 1-16

Inferior surface
R CORONARY ARTERY

Note: Most of the posterior portion of the heart as it lies rotated in
the chest becomes the _____ or _____ surface.   *inferior; diaphragmatic*
The right coronary artery is most significant for its blood supply

to the _____ wall of the _____ ventricle.   *inferoposterior   left*

IN SUMMARY:
The right coronary artery supplies the following:
1. S-A node (55%)
2. A-V node (90%)
3. bundle of His (a portion)
4. posteroinferior division of the left bundle (a portion)
5. posterior one-third of the septum
6. right atrial and ventricular muscle
7. inferoposterior wall of the left ventricle

The left coronary artery

74 The left coronary artery branches off from the _____ sinus of   *left*
Valsalva. It divides into two main branches as it reaches the surface of the heart—an *anterior descending* branch and a *lateral*
branch.

75 The anteriorly descending branch is called the _____   *anterior*

_____.   *descending*

CROSS SECTION   ANTERIOR   POSTERIOR
(AORTA)

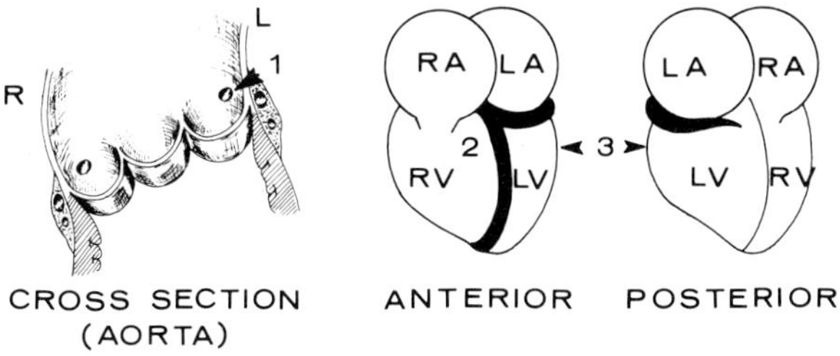

Fig. 1-17

The *anterior* descending gives off perforating branches from the
(front/back), which supply the *anterior two-thirds of the septum,*   *front*
a major portion of the *right bundle branch,* and the *anterosuperior*
division of the left bundle.

76 The lateral branch, called the *circumflex,* winds around the *(right/left)* side dividing the left atrium and the left ventricle anteriorly. This branch then travels around the back of the heart dividing the left atrium and left ventricle *(anteriorly/posteriorly).*   *left*

posteriorly

The circumflex may or may not descend, depending upon the individual. The circumflex supplies a portion of the posteroinferior division of the left bundle.

Note: The posteroinferior division has a dual blood supply—from both the right and the left coronary arteries.

77 The left coronary artery also supplies a portion of the cardiac

_____.   *muscle*

The left coronary artery divides into two main branches, the

_____ and the _____ _____   *circumflex;*
        anterior descending

The circumflex travels toward the *(right/left),* supplying the *lateral* portion of the left atrium and left ventricle.   *left*

The anterior descending descends _____ to supply the   *anteriorly*

_____ portion of the _____ ventricle.   *anterior   left*

The left coronary artery therefore supplies the _____ atrium and   *left*

the _____ portion of the left ventricle.   *anterolateral*

78 Let us again consider the left ventricle as it lies in the chest cavity:

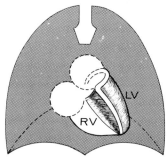

Fig. 1-18

L CORONARY ARTERY

The left coronary artery supplies a *(small/large)* portion of the left ventricle.   *large*

The left coronary artery is most significant because it provides the

blood supply to the _____ walls of the left ventricle.   *anterolateral*

IN SUMMARY:

Table 2. Left coronary artery

Anterior descending	*Circumflex*
1. Anterior ⅔ of septum	1. S-A node (45%)
2. Right bundle branch (RBB) (major portion)	2. Posteroinferior division of left bundle (a portion)
3. Anterosuperior division of left bundle	3. Lateral wall of left ventricle
4. Anterior wall of left ventricle	

79 Let us observe the interrelationship of the coronary arteries:

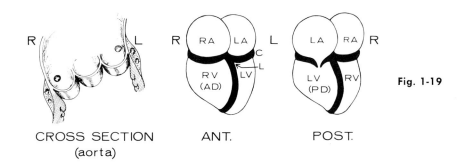

CROSS SECTION   ANT.   POST.   **Fig. 1-19**
    (aorta)

The ventricles are divided in the front by the _____ de-   *anterior*

scending branch of the _____ coronary artery.   *left*

The ventricles are divided in the back by the _____ de-   *posterior*

scending branch of the _____ coronary artery.   *right*

80 The right atrium and the right ventricle are divided anteriorly and

posteriorly by the _____ coronary artery.   *right*

The left atrium and the left ventricle are divided anteriorly and pos-

teriorly by the circumflex branch of the _____ coronary artery.   *left*

81 Let us again consider the left ventricle as it lies in the chest cavity:

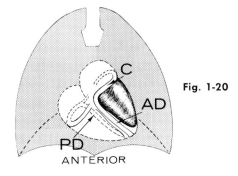

Fig. 1-20

82 **AD**—The anterior descending branch of the _____ coronary ar-   *left*

tery supplies the _____ wall of the left ventricle.   *anterior*

C—The circumflex branch of the _____ coronary artery supplies   *left*

the _____ wall of the left ventricle.   *lateral*

The left coronary artery as a whole supplies the _____   *anterolateral*

surface of the left ventricle.

83 **PD**—The inferoposterior portion of the left ventricle is supplied by

the _____ _____ branch of the _____ coronary   *posterior descending;*

artery.   *right*

The right coronary artery, then, supplies the _____posterior   *infero-*

portion of the left ventricle.

THE CORONARY VEINS

84 The heart receives its oxygenated blood via the coronary artery system. Deoxygenated blood returns to the heart via the *coronary veins.*

Like deoxygenated blood from the body, deoxygenated blood from

the heart itself empties into the _____ atrium.   *right*

85 The opening through which the coronary veins drain into the right
atrium is known as the *coronary sinus.*
The opening is located in the lower posterior portion of the right

_____.   *atrium*

86 IN SUMMARY:

Table 3. Coronary arteries

Right coronary artery supplies	*Left coronary artery supplies*
1. S-A node (55%)	1. S-A node (45%)
2. A-V node	2. Anterosuperior division of
3. Bundle of His (a portion)	left bundle
4. Posterior ⅓ of septum	3. Right bundle branch
5. Posteroinferior division of	(major portion)
left bundle (a portion)	4. Anterior ⅔ of septum
6. Inferoposterior surface of	5. Posteroinferior division of
left ventricle	left bundle (a portion)
	6. Anterolateral surface of left
	ventricle

The coronary veins return deoxygenated blood to the right atrium

via an opening known as the _____ _____.   *coronary sinus*

SUMMARY AND CORRELATION

87 The heart consists of a right side and a left side. The right and left
sides of the heart differ in:

1. _____   *function*

2. _____   *musculature*

3. _____ structure   *valvular*

88 *Let us review:*

Table 4

	Right ventricle	*Left ventricle*	*Right*	*Left*
A. *Function*				
	1. Delivers *unoxy-*	1. Delivers _____	body	oxygenated
	genated blood	blood from the		lungs
	from the _____	_____ to the	lungs	body
	to the _____.	_____.	lungs	body
	2. Projects its vol-	2. Projects its vol-		
	ume against	ume against		
	minimal resis-	maximum re-		
	tance—the	sistance—the		
	_____.	_____.		
B. *Musculature*				
	1. _____ walls	1. _____ walls	Thin	Thick
C. *Valvular structure*				
	1. *A-V valve:*	1. A-V valve:	tricuspid	mitral
	_____.	_____.		
	2. *Semilunar*	2. Semilunar	pulmonary	aortic
	valve: _____.	valve: _____.		

89 Within the chest wall the heart is _____ and positioned on *rotated*

its _____. *side*

The right ventricle therefore becomes the *(anterior/posterior)* ven- *anterior*
tricle.

The left ventricle becomes the *(anterior/posterior)* ventricle. *posterior*

Myocardial infarction occurs almost exclusively in the *(right/left)* *left*
ventricle.

In the setting of coronary care, the primary concern is therefore
the *(right/left)* ventricle. *left*

90 The heart has both _____ and _____ activity. *electrical   mechanical*

The *electrical activity* consists of:

    1. an electrical _____ (the initiating factor) *stimulus*

    2. _____ (the proliferating factor) *depolarization*

The electrical *properties* of the heart consist of:

    1. the ability to *initiate* an impulse (_____) *automaticity*

    2. the ability to *respond* to an impulse (_____) *excitability*

    3. the ability to *transmit* an impulse (_____) *conductivity*

91 The electrical activity of the heart is detected by the _____. *ECG*

Electrical activity of the heart begins in the _____ node, then *S-A*

continues on to the _____, _____ _____ _____, *atria; A-V junctional tissue; bundle of His; bundle branches; Purkinje fibers; ventricles*

_____ _____ _____, _____ _____, _____

_____, and _____.

The function of the electrical activity is to prepare the heart for

_____ activity. *mechanical*

92 The mechanical activity of the heart is known as _____. *contractility*

The mechanical activity of the heart is best detected by the _____. *pulse*
Mechanical activity of the heart begins with a period of contraction

or _____, followed by a period of relaxation or _____. *systole   diastole*

93 Mechanical activity enables the heart to function as a pump. The
amount of blood pumped from the heart is known as the cardiac

_____. *output*

Remember: Cardiac output is a product of _____ _____ *ventricular rate*

× _____ _____. *stroke volume*

94 Electrical activity prepares the heart for _____ activity. *mechanical*
Mechanical activity is the most important because it is the assur-

ance of actual _____ action. *pump*

For every beat on the ECG, there should be a corresponding

_____. *pulse*

95 Since *normal* heart function consists of normal _____ and *electrical*

_____ activity, *abnormal* heart function will result in dis- *mechanical*

turbances of either _____ activity, _____ activ- *electrical; mechanical*
ity, or both.

Abnormal *electrical* activity will result in arrhythmias.

Abnormal *mechanical* activity will result in heart failure or shock.

Suggested readings

Andreoli, K. G., and others: Comprehensive cardiac care, ed. 2, St. Louis, 1971, The C. V. Mosby Co.

Burrell, L., and Fuller, E. O.: Dissection of a beef heart with clinical correlations, Heart Lung 3 (4):643, July-Aug. 1974.

Ganong, W. F.: Review of medical physiology, Los Altos, Calif., 1969, Lange Medical Publications.

Gensimi, G. F., Buonanno, C., and Palacio, A.: Anatomy of the coronary circulation in living man, Dis. Chest 52:125, 1967.

Gould, S. E., editor: Pathology of the heart and blood vessels, Springfield, Ill., 1968, Charles C Thomas, Publisher.

Guyton, A. C.: Textbook of medical physiology, Philadelphia, 1971, W. B. Saunders Co.

Hurst, W. J., and Logue, R. B., editors: The heart arteries and veins, New York, 1970, McGraw-Hill Book Co.

James, T.: The coronary circulation and conduction system, Prog. Cardiov. Dis. 10:410, 1968.

Netter, F. H.: Heart—The Ciba Collection of Medical Illustrations, Summit, N. J., 1969, Ciba Publications.

Pansky, B., and House, E. L.: Review of gross anatomy, London, 1969, The Macmillan Co.

Rosenbaum, M. B., Elizari, M. V., and Lazzari, J. O.: The hemiblocks, Oldsmar, Fla., 1970, Tampa Tracings.

Schamroth, L.: An introduction to electrocardiography, Edinburgh, 1971, Blackwell Scientific Publications.

Warner, H. F., Russell, M. W., and Spann, J. F.: Heart muscle: Clinical applications of basic physiology and cellular anatomy, Heart Lung 1 (4):464, July-Aug. 1972.

Basic electrophysiology

In Unit 1 it was stated that the heart has both electrical and mechanical properties. The heart has the *electrical* ability to: (1) *initiate* electrical impulses (automaticity); (2) *respond* to electrical impulses (excitability); (3) *conduct* electrical impulses (conductivity). The heart also has the *mechanical* ability to respond to these impulses with pump action (contractility).

CONDUCTION

1 The heart's electrical impulses are transmitted or conducted by the process of *depolarization.* At rest, the electrical system is negatively charged, or *polarized.* (See Unit 3.)

The advancing electrical impulse causes a movement of positive charges into the cells. The inside of these cells now becomes *(electropositive/electronegative)* and the cells are said to be *electropositive*

_____. *depolarized*

Depolarization may be described as an advancing wave of *(positive/ positive* *negative)* charges.

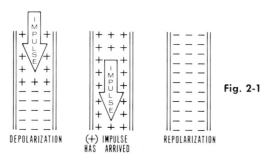

Fig. 2-1

DEPOLARIZATION   (+) IMPULSE   REPOLARIZATION
HAS ARRIVED

The movement of positive charges into the myocardial cells causes

them to become _____. *depolarized*
After the impulse has left, the electrical system is again recharged,

or _____. *repolarized*

2 Let us review the normal sequence of conduction:

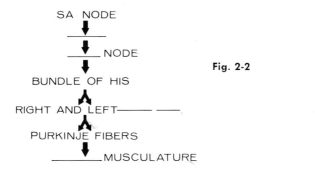

Fig. 2-2

SA NODE

_____   *atria*

_____ NODE   *A-V*

BUNDLE OF HIS

RIGHT AND LEFT_____ ___   *bundle branches*

PURKINJE FIBERS

_____ MUSCULATURE   *ventricular*

Note: The conduction system in the heart may be compared to a rapid transit system. It provides the most rapid means for the transmission of an electrical impulse. If there is a block in this system (for example, S-A block, A-V block, or bundle branch block), the heart can still be depolarized, but the process will occur more slowly.

THE NORMAL ECG COMPLEX

3 The wave of depolarization and repolarization spreading through the heart can be recorded on paper. This record is called the electrocardiogram, or ECG.

Let us analyze the normal configuration of the ECG:

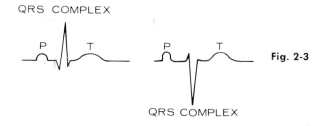

Fig. 2-3

4 The electrical impulses spreading through the atria produce the *P wave.*

The P wave represents depolarization of the _____.

atria

The electrical impulses spreading through the ventricles produce the QRS complex. The QRS complex, therefore, represents depolarization of the _____.

ventricles

5 Let us consider the QRS complex in more detail: a *Q wave* is defined as the first negative deflection in the QRS complex.

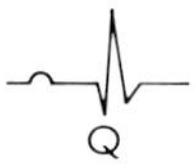

Fig. 2-4

In Fig. 2-4 there *(is/is not)* a Q wave.

is

Remember: A Q wave is defined as the first *(positive/negative)* deflection in the complex.

negative

The *R wave* is defined as the first positive deflection in the complex. The *S wave* is defined as the first negative deflection occurring after the R wave.

6 Consider this QRS complex:

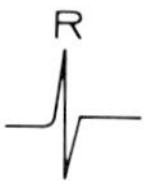

Fig. 2-5

The first deflection is *(positive/negative).* It is called the _____ wave. The second deflection is *(positive/negative).* It is called the _____ wave. In this complex, there *(is/is not)* a Q wave.

positive   R
negative
S   *is not*

7 Every QRS *complex* does not always have a Q, an R, and an S. However, the wave representing ventricular depolarization is collectively

known as the *QRS complex*, regardless of its configuration. All QRS
complexes *(do/do not)* have a Q, an R, and an S.

do not

All QRS complexes do reflect _____ depolarization.

ventricular

8 Each wave in the QRS complex may be further described according
to its *size*. A large wave would be denoted by a capital letter—Q, R,
or S. A small wave would be denoted by a small letter—*q*, *r*, or *s*.
Label the following complexes:

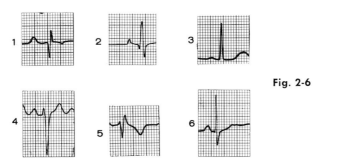

Fig. 2-6

1. *QR*

2. *qRs*

3. *R*

4. *rS*

5. *rSr'*

6. *Rs*

Note: In 5, there is a second positive deflection. When this occurs,
the wave is labeled *R prime* or *R'*.
Remember: Q waves and S waves are always *(positive/negative)*.

negative

R waves are always _____.

positive

9 After depolarization has occurred, the heart must recover before
it can receive another impulse. This process is known as

_____.

repolarization

Ventricular repolarization is represented on the ECG by the *T wave*.
Atrial repolarization is also represented by a T wave. However, this
impulse is usually not seen on the ECG because it is hidden within
the QRS complex and is of low voltage.
Note: Identification of both the T wave and P wave may be facilitated by *first* identifying the large and more distinct QRS complex
and using it as a guide.

THE INTERVALS OF THE ECG COMPLEX

10 Certain *intervals* on the ECG are also significant. The first to be
considered is the *P-R interval*. It is measured from the beginning
of the P wave to the beginning of the QRS complex.

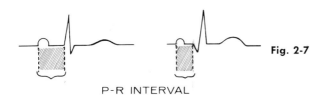

Fig. 2-7

P-R INTERVAL

Note: In Fig. 2-7 the second interval is actually a p-q interval.
The P-R interval begins with atrial depolarization and ends with

the *beginning* of _____ depolarization. It represents the
delay between atrial and ventricular depolarization, or the time

ventricular

that it takes an impulse to travel from the _____ node to the

S-A

_____. It serves to correlate the electrical impulse of the   *ventricles*
atria with that of the ventricle. The normal P-R interval is from
0.12 to 0.20 second.
A P-R interval of constant duration serves to establish a constant

relationship between _____ and _____.   *P   QRS*

11 Another frequently measured interval in electrocardiography is the
Q-T interval.

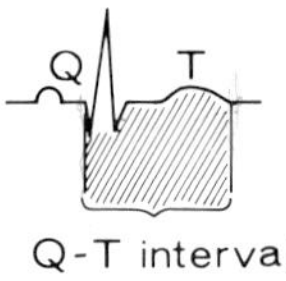

Fig. 2-8

Q-T interval

The Q-T interval includes ventricular depolarization (the QRS

complex) plus ventricular _____, or the _____ wave.   *repolarization   T*

12 Let us now consider a specific portion of the Q-T interval, the *QRS*

duration. The QRS complex represents _____   *ventricular*

_____. The QRS is measured from the beginning of the   *depolarization*
Q wave to the end of the S wave. The normal QRS duration is from
0.08 to 0.12 second.
Note: If there is no Q wave present, the "QRS" is measured from
the beginning of the first deflection in the complex.

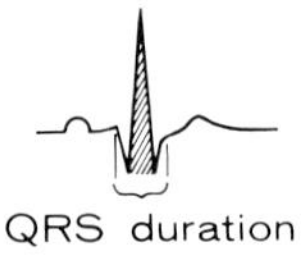

Fig. 2-9

QRS duration

13 Another important interval within the Q-T interval is called the
S-T segment. The "j" or junction point marks the beginning of the
segment. The S-T segment represents the heart's resting period between *(atrial/ventricular)* depolarization and repolarization.   *ventricular*

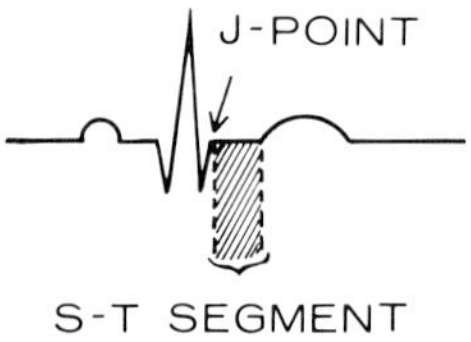

J-POINT

Fig. 2-10

S-T SEGMENT

THE REFRACTORY PERIODS

14 During the depolarization and repolarization the heart has periods
of varying excitability. These periods are known as the *refractory
periods.*
Remember: Excitability is the ability of the heart to _____   *respond*
to an electrical impulse.
Therefore, the refractory periods of the heart are times during
which its ability to respond to an electrical impulse varies.
The refractory periods of the ventricles are represented by certain
areas within the Q-T interval:

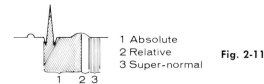

1 Absolute
2 Relative
3 Super-normal

Fig. 2-11

15 The absolute refractory period is that time during the cardiac cycle when the heart will not respond to any stimuli. An electrical stimulus reaching the ventricles during the absolute refractory period *(will/will not)* cause a myocardial response.

will not

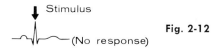

Stimulus

Fig. 2-12

(No response)

In the normal heart, the *absolute* refractory period includes the

QRS and part of the _____ segment.

S-T why not just the T?

16 The *relative* refractory period is that time during the cardiac cycle when only a *strong* stimulus can cause a response.

17 The *supernormal* period is that time during the cardiac cycle when a *weak* stimulus can cause a response.

18 The *vulnerable* period is that portion of the cardiac cycle when a stimulus of *any* strength may cause repetitive firing. In the setting of acute myocardial infarction, the vulnerable period usually occurs on the *apex* of the T wave.

Any stimulus that occurs during the *vulnerable* period of the cardiac cycle may cause *repetitive firing*. This response is analogous to a chain reaction.

Let us review:

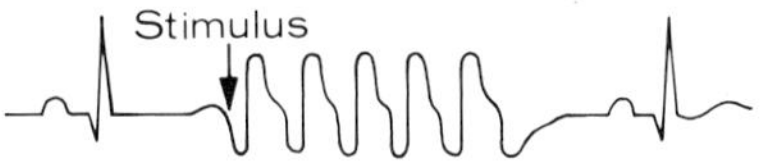

Stimulus

Fig. 2-13

19 During the *absolute* refractory period, the heart *(will/will not)* respond to any stimulus.

will not

During the *relative* refractory period, a *(weak/strong)* stimulus may elicit a response.

strong

During the *supernormal* period, a *(weak/strong)* stimulus may elicit a response.

weak

During the vulnerable period, a stimulus of any intensity may cause

_____ _____.

repetitive firing

In the setting of acute myocardial infarction, the vulnerable period

ocurs on the apex of the _____ wave.

T

THE ELECTROCARDIOGRAM

20 Before discussing the normal electrocardiogram, we must first consider the derivation of leads. A lead is composed of a *negative* and a *positive* electrode. These electrodes "sense" electricity. The movement of electricity in the heart may be sensed by a _____. A lead

lead

is composed of a _____ electrode and a _____ elec-   *negative*   *positive*
trode.

Note: When the positive and negative electrodes are both located
on the body's surface, this is known as a *bipolar* lead. When the
positive electrode is located on the body surface and the negative
electrode is in infinity, this is known as a *unipolar* lead.

The limb leads

21 A *standardized* method of electrode placement was devised by Einthoven.

In devising this method, he first considered the *frontal plane*. The
frontal plane corresponds to an *anterior* view of the patient.

Remember: The borders of the frontal plane are:

1. _____   *right*

2. _____   *left*

3. _____   *superior*

4. _____   *inferior*

22 Positions on the arms and legs were selected as electrode sites:

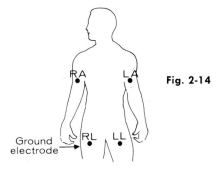

Fig. 2-14

Note: These limb positions border the _____ plane.   *frontal*
Using two electrodes at a time, three bipolar leads were derived.

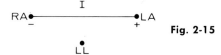

Fig. 2-15

23 Using the two arm electrodes, the left arm **(LA)** is made positive
and the right arm **(RA)** is made negative. This is known as *Lead I*
(Fig. 2-15).

In Lead I, the positive electrode is on the _____ arm.   *left*

In Lead I, the negative electrode is on the _____ arm.   *right*

24 Using the right arm electrode **(RA)** and the foot electrode **(F)**, the
right arm is made negative and the foot is made positive. This is
known as *Lead II*.

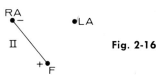

Fig. 2-16

In Lead II, the positive electrode is at the _____.

foot

In Lead II, the negative electrode is on the _____ arm.

right

25 Using the left arm (**LA**) and the foot (**F**) electrodes, the left arm is made negative and the foot is made positive. This is known as *Lead III*.

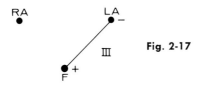

Fig. 2-17

In Lead III, the positive electrode is at the _____.

foot

In Lead III, the negative electrode is on the _____ arm.

left

26 *Note:* The right leg (**RL**) serves as the ground electrode for these leads.

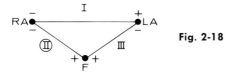

Fig. 2-18

Fig. 2-18 summarizes the three bipolar leads.

27 Three more angles, or leads, from which to record information in the frontal plane were derived. Each electrode on the body was made *positive*, and the *negative* electrode was extended to infinity.
Remember: When the positive electrode is on the body surface and

the negative electrode is at infinity, this is called a _____ lead.

unipolar

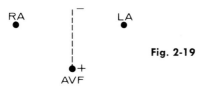

Fig. 2-19

28 Lead aVF was created by making the foot electrode positive and extending the negative electrode to infinity.
It takes more electrical energy to allow the negative electrode to exist in infinity. This extra energy is known as *augmented voltage*. For this reason, this lead is known as the augmented voltage foot lead or *Lead aVF*.
In Lead aVF, the positive electrode is at the _____. In Lead aVF,

foot

the negative electrode is at _____. Lead aVF has *(one/two)* visible electrode(s) on the body. It is therefore called a *(unipolar/ bipolar)* lead.

infinity   *one*

unipolar

29 Using the same principles, the RA and LA electrodes were used to obtain *Leads aVR and aVL*.

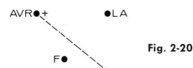

Fig. 2-20

In *Lead aVR*, the positive electrode is on the right arm, and the negative electrode is at _____.

infinity

30

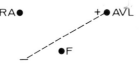

Fig. 2-21

In *Lead aVL*, the positive electrode is on the *(left/right)* arm and the negative electrode is at _____.

left

31 Fig. 2-22 is a representation of all the limb leads.

infinity

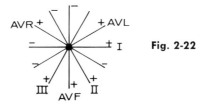

Fig. 2-22

32 Let us analyze how this diagram was derived.

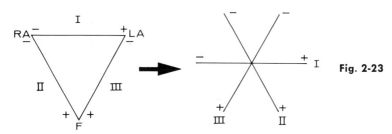

Fig. 2-23

The three *bipolar* limb leads are _____, _____, and _____. They may be moved to a center point so that they intersect. The heart may be pictured in the center as in Fig. 2-24.

I   II   III

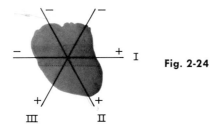

Fig. 2-24

33 Let us add the three unipolar limb leads, _____, _____, and _____.

aVR   aVL
aVF

28

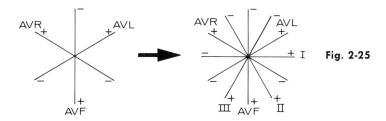

Fig. 2-25

Correlation

34 Let us consider the forces of the heart in relationship to the leads. In the normal heart, the *(right/left)* ventricle has the most *muscle mass* and the most *electrical forces.*

    left

For this reason, the sum of all the electrical forces traveling through the ventricles is usually a force shifted slightly to the *left.*

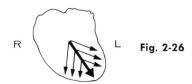

Fig. 2-26

35 In Fig. 2-26, the arrows represent both *magnitude* and *direction* of force. These arrows are known as *vectors.*

The summation force (large arrow) is known as the summation

_____ or *axis.*

    vector

36 The ventricular, or QRS, axis in the normal heart is shifted toward the *(right/left).*

    left

Note: An axis can also be derived for both the P wave and T wave. However, when discussing *the* axis of the heart, we are usually considering the axis of the *QRS complex.*

It is the ventricular axis, or ventricular summation *vector,* that is

reflected on the ECG as the _____ complex.

    QRS

37 Electrical forces traveling toward a positive electrode produce a positive deflection on the ECG.

Electrical forces traveling toward a negative electrode or away

from a positive pole produce a _____ deflection on the ECG.

    negative

38 Einthoven designated the polarity for Lead I:

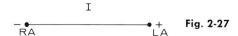

Fig. 2-27

By superimposing the ventricular forces of a particular patient's heart over Lead I, we can deduce the morphology of his QRS in this lead:

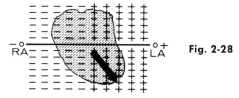

Fig. 2-28

29

The ventricular forces of this patient *(are/are not)* traveling in a normal direction.

are

39 The ventricular forces of this person's normal heart travel *(toward/ away from)* the positive electrode in Lead I. Therefore, it can be expected that a normal QRS complex in Lead I will have a predominantly *(positive/negative)* deflection.

toward

positive

Lead I

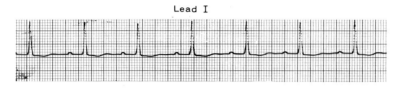

Fig. 2-29

40 In Lead II, this patient's ventricular forces also travel toward the positive electrode.

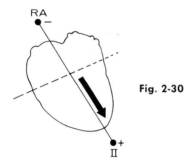

Fig. 2-30

Therefore the normal QRS in Lead II will have a *(positive/negative)* deflection.

positive

41 *Remember:* On the ECG, the P wave represents the atrial electrical forces, or the P wave axis.
The normal forces of the atria also travel toward the positive electrode in Lead II.
In Lead II, therefore, the P wave is also *(positive/negative)*.
It can be expected that, during normal conduction, P waves will be

positive

upright and best visible in lead _____.

II

42 Using these principles of electrophysiology, we can deduce the QRS morphology in all of the limb leads.
Review Fig. 2-31, below.

43 In Lead aVR, the normal QRS complex should be predominantly *(positive/negative)*.

negative

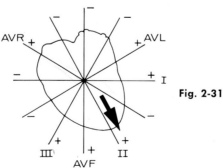

Fig. 2-31

The P wave in Lead aVR is also negative, because the atrial forces are moving *(toward/away from)* the positive electrode.   *away from*

Remember: The normal P wave is always positive in Lead _____   *II*

and always negative in Lead _____. Therefore, P waves are best   *aVR*
identified in these two leads.

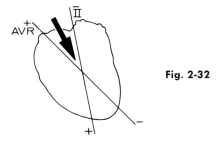

Fig. 2-32

44 Let us now examine the six-lead ECG and verify the configuration
of all of the limb leads:

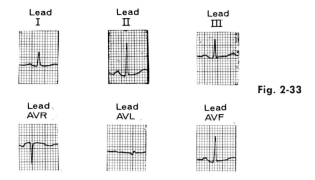

Fig. 2-33

Remember: The major direction of the QRS deflection is determined by both the direction of the ventricular forces and the po-

sition of the positive _____ of each lead.   *electrode*

The chest leads

45 The limb leads provide six views of the heart in the *frontal plane.*
Another view of the heart's electrical activity can be seen in the
horizontal plane. This plane is obtained by viewing a person trans-
versely, anteriorly, and posteriorly.

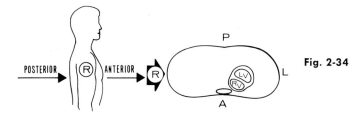

Fig. 2-34

46 The *V leads,* or *chest leads,* provide six possible views of the heart
in the *horizontal* plane.
The V leads were derived using the principle of the unipolar leads.
They also represent augmented voltage of vector forces and thus
are known as V leads.

In the V leads, the positive electrode is placed on the chest wall and the negative electrode is extended to _____.

infinity

47 The positive electrode of V_1 is located just to the right of the sternum in the fourth intercostal space. The positive electrode is then moved along the chest wall toward the left to form leads V_2, V_3, V_4, V_5, and V_6.

48

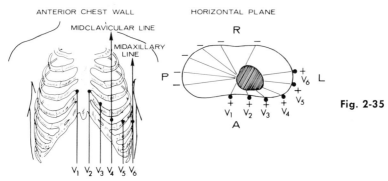

ELECTRODE POSITION

Fig. 2-35

The positive electrodes in all of the chest leads are located on the front and side of the chest. The negative electrodes are located toward the back at _____.

infinity

49 The forces of the QRS axis travel toward the *(right/left)* ventricle. The left ventricle lies rotated *posteriorly* in the chest. Therefore, the QRS forces in the horizontal plane travel *(anteriorly/posteriorly)*.

left

posteriorly

50 Using this information, the normal QRS direction in the chest leads can be deduced.
In Lead V_1, the QRS forces travel toward the *(positive/negative)* electrode. Therefore, the normal QRS in Lead V_1 should be predominantly *(positive/negative)*.
In Lead V_6, the QRS forces travel toward the *(positive/negative)* electrode. Therefore, the normal QRS in Lead V_6 should be predominantly *(positive/negative)*.

negative

negative
positive

positive

51 *Note:* Leads V_2 to V_5 are a transition from the V_1 pattern to the V_6 pattern. The R wave becomes larger and the S wave smaller as the progression occurs.
Let us examine the chest leads of the ECG in Fig. 2-36 to verify these configurations:

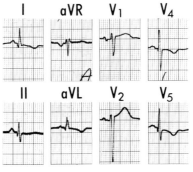
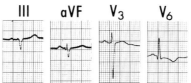

Fig. 2-36

52 To complete a study of QRS configurations, we must consider the force created by depolarization of the septum. This force, though small, contributes to the QRS complex.

The septum is the first portion of the ventricle to be depolarized. Septal depolarization occurs from left to right and posteriorly to anteriorly. *Remember:* The ventricles are depolarized from right to

_____ and _____ to posteriorly. Thus, septal depolariza-   *left*   *anteriorly*
tion ocurs in the *(same/opposite)* direction.   *opposite*

Therefore, it can be expected that the initial part of the QRS complex will have a small *opposite* deflection.

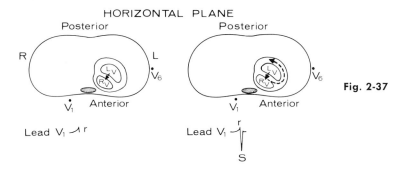

Fig. 2-37

53 In *Lead V_1* in Fig. 2-37 the initial, or septal, force is represented by a *small r* wave. This is caused by the wave of septal depolarization traveling toward the *(right/left)*.   *right*

The *major* ventricular forces travel in the *(same/opposite)* direction, toward the *(right/left)*.   *opposite*
                   left

In Lead V_1, this force is represented by a large *(R/S)* wave.   *S*

54 In *Lead V_6* in Fig. 2-38 the initial, or septal, force is represented by a *small q* wave. This is caused by the wave of septal depolarization traveling *(toward/away from)* V_6.   *away from*

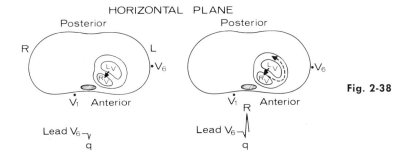

Fig. 2-38

The *major* ventricular forces travel in the *(same/opposite)* direction, producing a large *(R/S)* wave in Lead V_6.   *opposite*
                   R

55 Let us now consider the surfaces of the left ventricle and correlate the *leads* and the area of *electrical activity* which each reflects.

Electrical forces of the heart are recorded as they travel toward or away from the *(positive/negative)* electrode. Therefore the *positive* electrode may be considered the most sensitive electrode.   *positive*

56 The foot electrode looks directly toward the *(inferior/anterior)* surface of the left ventricle. The leads that use the foot as a positive   *inferior*

electrode are Leads _____, _____, and _____.   *II*   *III*   *aVF*

Leads II, III, and aVF, then, reflect the electrical activity of the

_____ surface of the left ventricle. Therefore, inferior wall   *inferior*

myocardial infarctions (IWMI) can best be detected in Leads _____,   *II*

_____, and _____.   *III   aVF*

Consider the relationship of these leads to the inferior wall:

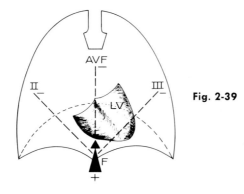

Fig. 2-39

57   Let us now discuss the *anterior* surface and the leads that reflect
its electrical activity.
The left arm electrode (LA) looks directly at the *lateral* portion of
the anterior surface of the left ventricle. The leads that use the left

arm as the positive electrode are Leads _____ and _____.   *I   aVL*

Leads I and aVL, then, reflect the _____ surface of the left   *lateral*
ventricle.

58   The positive electrodes of the *chest leads* look at the septal and
lateral portion of the anterior surface of the left ventricle.
Therefore, Leads I, aVL, and V_1 to V_6 reflect the electrical activity

of the entire _____ wall.   *anterior*
It can then be expected that extensive anterior wall myocardial in-

farctions (AWMI) will best be seen in Leads _____ and _____ and   *I   aVL*
in the *(chest/limb)* leads.   *chest*

59   Consider the anterior wall in Fig. 2-40.

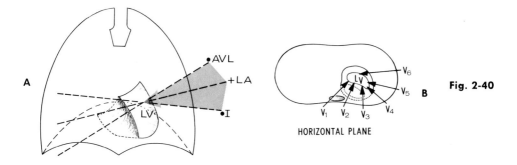

HORIZONTAL PLANE

Fig. 2-40

Note: If an infarction is confined to the *septal* area of the anterior
wall it is best seen in Leads V_1 to V_4. If an infarction is confined
to the lateral portion of the anterior wall, it is best seen in Leads I,
aVL, and V_4 to V_6.

60 An acute injury current in the *lateral* leads will produce opposite, or *reciprocal*, changes in the _____ leads, which are _____, _____, and _____.

inferior   II

III   aVF

An acute injury current in the *inferior* leads will produce opposite, or *reciprocal*, changes in the _____ leads, which are _____, _____, and V_4 to V_6.

lateral   I

aVL

An acute injury in the anteroseptal area will produce no reciprocal changes in any of the standard leads because there are no standard electrode positions directly opposite it.

61 Let us now consider *Lead aVR* and its relationship to the left ventricle:

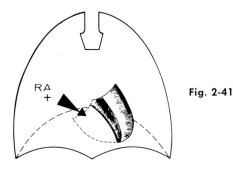

Fig. 2-41

Lead aVR uses the RA as its *(positive/negative)* electrode. The RA electrode does not look directly at any *surface* of the left ventricle. This lead, however, does look at the *inside* of the heart. Lead aVR reflects the *(outside/inside)* of the left ventricle. Lead aVR is known as an *intracavitary lead*.

positive

inside

SINUS RHYTHMS

62 A sinus rhythm is one that originates in the sinus node.
Let us review the conduction of a sinus impulse:

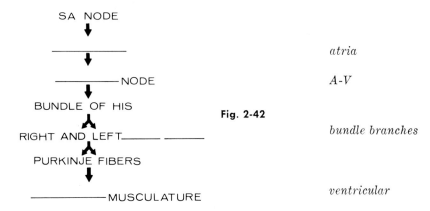

Fig. 2-42

atria

A-V

bundle branches

ventricular

63 *When interpreting rhythms,* we suggest that the following systematic approach be used:
1. Analyze the QRS complex
2. Analyze the P wave
3. Analyze the relationship between the P wave and the QRS complex (P-R interval)

64 Sinus rhythm is diagnosed according to the following criteria:
1. QRS complex—narrow and unchanging
2. P wave—visible preceding each QRS complex; upright (in Lead
   II); no sudden irregularities in p-p interval; P wave rate 150 or
   less
3. P-R interval—a QRS complex follows each P wave at constant
   intervals of normal duration.

65 The most flexible of these criteria is the width of the QRS complex.
Sinus rhythm can occur in the presence of an abnormal or wide
QRS. Width implies that there is delay. A wide QRS occurring in a
constant relationship with a normal P wave (as evidenced by a constant p-r interval) means that the normal sinus impulse has been

_____ in the ventricles.   *delayed*
Sinus rhythm can be diagnosed from a normal P wave alone, since
this implies the impulse is of normal atrial origin (the S-A node).
A constant P-R interval of normal duration serves to verify that the
sinus impulse is conducted normally.

66 *Let us review:* Sinus rhythm usually has a narrow and _____   *unchanging*
QRS, a P wave that is *(positive/negative)* in Lead II, and a P-R   *positive*

interval that is constant and of _____ duration.   *normal*

67 After the origin of a rhythm has been identified as sinus, it is fur-

ther classified according to discharge sequence, or _____ wave rate.   *P*

ATRIAL RATE

NORMAL SINUS RHYTHM	60—100	
SINUS BRADYCARDIA	LESS THAN 60	**Fig. 2-43**
SINUS TACHYCARDIA	101 — 150	

In sinus rhythm the atrial rate and the ventricular rate are usually
the same, so the P wave rate will correspond to the more easily
measured QRS rate.

68 Measurement of ventricular rate is made from one QRS complex to
the next QRS complex.
Note: When measuring ventricular rate, any component of the
QRS may be used as reference point. However, the measurement
must be made between two consistent points, that is, R-R, q-q, s-s.

69 Let us now discuss the calculation of ventricular rates.
ECG paper is divided by markings into intervals that represent
spans of 3 seconds. (See Fig. 2-44, p. 37).
The ventricular rate for 1 minute may be estimated rapidly by
counting the number of R waves occurring in a 6-second time span
and *multiplying* this number by 10. This will give the number of R

waves occurring in 60 seconds, the _____ rate for 1 min-   *ventricular*
ute.

70 The ventricular rate may also be obtained by multiplying the num-

ber of R waves occurring in one 3-second span by _____. This will   *20*
also give the ventricular rate for 1 minute.

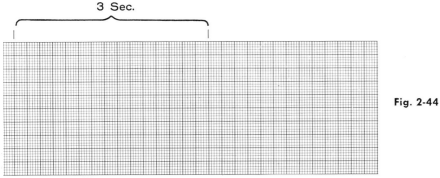

3 Sec.

Fig. 2-44

71 Estimate the ventricular rate in the following 6-second ECG strip:

The ventricular rate is approximately _____.   *70*

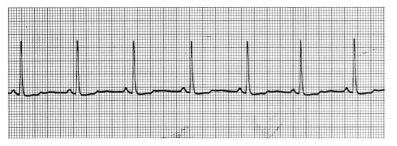

Fig. 2-45

72 A more accurate method for estimating rates has also been devised. We suggest that the student follow these steps when calculating rates: (1) obtain an ECG rhythm strip; (2) look for an R wave that falls on a dark line or at the beginning of a larger box. The rate will be estimated from this point—consider this R wave to be a *reference point.*

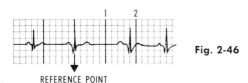

Fig. 2-46

REFERENCE POINT

73 Each dark line occurring after the "R wave reference point" has been assigned a value. Therefore, it is necessary for the student to memorize the values of each subsequent line:

Line	Value
1	300
2	150
3	100
4	75
5	60
6	50
7	43
8	37
9	33

74 Consider this ECG strip:

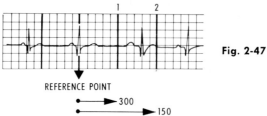

Fig. 2-47

REFERENCE POINT

Note: On an ECG graph recording at a standard paper speed of 25 mm per second each large box (between two dark lines) = 0.20 second. Each small box (between two light colored lines) = 0.04 second. Therefore, if a QRS complex occurs on every dark line, it means a ventricular impulse is occurring every 0.20 second, or 300 times per minute (60 sec./min. ÷ 0.20 sec./beat).

75 The ventricular rate can be estimated as follows: If an R wave falls on the first dark line that occurs *after* the reference point, the value

is 300, and the ventricular rate then equals _____ beats per minute.　　*300*
If an R wave falls on the second dark line occurring after the ref-

erence point, the value is _____ and the ventricular rate is then　　*150*

_____ beats per minute.　　*150*

Note: Ventricular rate is measured *between two points, or beats.* The first is the "R wave reference point" and the second is the very next occurring beat.

76 Practice estimating ventricular rates:

The ventricular rate (Fig. 2-48) is _____.　　*100*

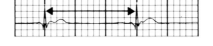

Fig. 2-48

The ventricular rate (Fig. 2-49) is _____.　　*75*

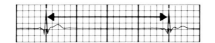

Fig. 2-49

77 Note that each large box is composed of five smaller boxes. These smaller components must be considered when calculating rates that fall between the preassigned values.
Look at this example:

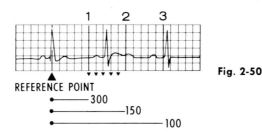

Fig. 2-50

REFERENCE POINT

78 The first complex that occurs after the reference point is located

between line __ and line __. *Remember:* Line 1 = 300 and line 2 =　　*1　　2*

150. Therefore, the ventricular rate in this example falls between

_____ and _____ beats per minute. The rate is *(less than/*   *150   300*

greater than) 150, and is *(less than/greater than)* 300.   *greater than;*

                                                            less than

79 To obtain the value of the space between these two lines, *subtraction* is used.

$$\text{In Fig. 2-50: Line 1} = 300$$
$$\text{Line 2} = \underline{150}$$
$$150$$

So there are 150 unit values between line 1 and line 2.

80 *Remember:* There are five smaller boxes within each large box *or* between two dark lines. To obtain the value of each small box, division is used.

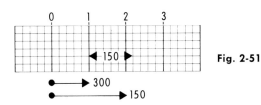

Fig. 2-51

In Fig. 2-51:

$$\text{Between line 1 and 2} = \frac{150}{} = 30$$
$$\text{Number of small boxes} = \overline{5}$$

Each small box then equals _____.   *30*

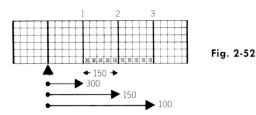

Fig. 2-52

$$\text{Between line 2 and 3} = \frac{50 \text{ (rate difference)}}{} = 10$$
$$\text{Number of small boxes} = \overline{5}$$

81 Evaluate this practice strip:

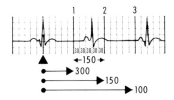

Fig. 2-53

The first complex after the reference point falls between lines 1 and

2. The rate must therefore be between _____ and _____ beats per   *150   300*

minute. Each small square = _____.   *30*

82 The second complex falls on the second small box past 150. Therefore the rate would be *(greater than/less than)* 150 per minute.   *greater than*

Two small boxes = 2 × 30 = _____. Add this number to the value   *60*
of line 2.

$$\begin{array}{ll} \text{Line 2} & = 150 \\ \text{Small boxes} & = +60 \\ \hline & 210 \end{array}$$

The ventricular rate, then, is _____ beats per minute.   *210*

83 When interpreting the ECG strip, the *P-R interval* must also be
measured.
The P-R interval is measured from the beginning of the _____ wave   *P*

to the beginning of the _____ _____.   *QRS complex*
Remember: The P-R interval extends from the beginning of

_____ depolarization to the beginning of _____ depo-   *atrial; ventricular*
larization.

84 On graph paper, one large box = *0.20 second*. Each large box is di-

vided into five smaller boxes. Therefore, each small box = _____   *0.04*
second.
To determine the P-R interval, the number of small boxes occurring
during the period is multipled by 0.04 second.

85 Look at this example:

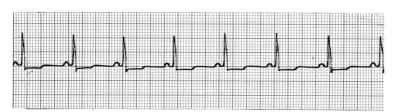

Fig. 2-54

Using the second complex from the end as clearest, the number of
small boxes in the P-R interval = 3. The P-R interval here =

_____ second.   *0.12*

Note: The normal P-R interval is from 0.12 to 0.20 second.

Suggested readings

Dubin, D.: Rapid interpretation of EKG's, Tampa, Fla., 1970, Cover Publishing Co.

Ganong, W. F.: Review of medical physiology, Los Altos, Calif., 1969, Lange Medical Publications.

Guyton, A. C.: Textbook of medical physiology, Philadelphia, 1971, W. B. Saunders Co.

Hurst, W. J., and Logue, R. B., editors: The heart arteries and veins, New York, 1970, McGraw-Hill Book Co.

Mariott, H. T.: Practical electrocardiography, Baltimore, 1968, The Williams & Wilkins Co.

Netter, F. H.: Heart—The Ciba Collection of Medical Illustrations, Summit, N. J., 1969, Ciba Publications.

Schamroth, L.: An introduction to electrocardiography, Edinburgh, 1971, Blackwell Scientific Publications.

Scherf, D.: Remarks on the nomenclature of cardiac arrhythmias, Prog. Cardiov. Dis. 13:1, 1970.

Winsor, T.: The electrocardiogram in myocardial infarction, Summit, N. J., 1968, Ciba Publications.

The chemical imbalances

FLUID AND ELECTROLYTE BALANCE
Definitions

1 The body's fluid is located within two major compartments.
Intracellular fluid (ICF) is located *(inside/outside)* the cell.   *inside*
Extracellular fluid (ECF) is located *(inside/outside)* the cell.   *outside*
The extracellular fluid includes intravascular and interstitial fluid.
Intravascular fluid (IVF) is within the blood vesels.
Interstitial fluid (ISF) is located between the cells and the blood vessels.

Extracellular fluid is made up of _____ fluid and   *intravascular*

_____ fluid.   *interstitial*

2 IN SUMMARY:

IVF   ICF
ISF
ICF   **Fig. 3-1**
BLOOD VESSELS   CELLS

3 *Ions* are electrically charged particles contained within the body fluid compartments. An *anion* is a negatively charged particle. The two main anions in the body are chloride (Cl^-) and bicarbonate (HCO_3^-).
A *cation* is a positively charged particle. The three main cations in the body are potassium (K^+), sodium (Na^+), and calcium (Ca^{++}).
An electrolyte is a combination of an anion and a cation in solution, which when dissolved in water will conduct an electrical current. Examples of electrolytes are sodium chloride ($NaCl$) and potassium chloride (KCl).
A cation has a *(positive/negative)* charge.   *positive*
An anion has a *(positive/negative)* charge.   *negative*

KCl is an example of an _____.   *electrolyte*

The anion in KCl is _____.   *Cl^-*

The cation in KCl is _____.   *K^+*

4 *Diffusion* is the movement of particles from a region of greater concentration to a region of lesser concentration. An example of diffusion is the gaseous exchange in the lungs.

Oxygen (particles) moves from a region of _____ concentra-   *greater*

tion (the air) to a region of _____ concentration (venous blood).   *lesser*

5 *Osmosis* is the movement of water from a region of lesser concentration (of dissolved particles) to a region of greater concentration

41

(of dissolved particles). Within the body cells semipermeable membranes limit the free movement of some particles. In this setting

the movement of fluid via the process of _____ aids in sta-   *osmosis*
bilizing fluid concentration.

6 IN SUMMARY:

DIFFUSION	OSMOSIS
MOVEMENT OF PARTICLES	MOVEMENT OF WATER
GREATER TO LESSER CONCENTRATION	LESSER TO GREATER CONCENTRATION
EXAMPLE: GASEOUS EXCHANGE IN THE LUNGS	EXAMPLE: WATER TRANSPORT IN THE CELLS.

Fig. 3-2

Remember: Osmosis is the movement of _____. In osmosis, move-   *water*

ment occurs from a region of _____ concentration to a region of   *lesser*

_____ concentration of dissolved particles.   *greater*

7 A *hypotonic* solution is one with a lesser concentration of dissolved particles.
A *hypertonic* solution is one with a greater concentration of dissolved particles.

8 Let us consider *osmosis* in more detail:

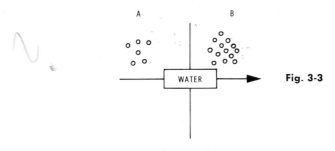

Fig. 3-3

In Fig. 3-3: Solution A is _____ in relation to Solution   *hypotonic*

B; Solution B is _____ in relation to Solution A.   *hypertonic*

9 During osmosis, water moves from the more dilute, or

_____, solution to the more concentrated, or   *hypotonic*

_____, solution. This represents an effort to equalize the   *hypertonic*
concentrations of both solutions. This body is continuously striving toward a state of equilibrium, or *homeostasis*.
The process of osmosis is an attempt to maintain _____.   *homeostasis*

10 Let us consider Solution A to be the serum (blood) and Solution B to be a *cell:*

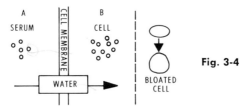

Fig. 3-4

In Fig. 3-4, the serum is *(hypotonic/hypertonic)*. Water therefore moves from the _____ into the _____; the cells then become _____.

hypotonic

serum   cell

bloated

11 If the situation is reversed, Solution A would represent a *cell* and Solution B the *serum:*

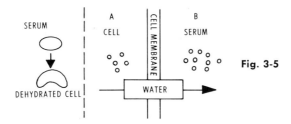

SERUM

DEHYDRATED CELL

A
CELL

CELL MEMBRANE

B
SERUM

WATER

Fig. 3-5

In Fig. 3-5, the serum is *(hypertonic/hypotonic)*. Water moves from the _____ into the _____. The cells become _____.

hypertonic
cells; serum;
*   dehydrated*

12 Hypertonic solutions "pull" water *(into/out of)* the cells. Mannitol and 50% glucose are examples of hypertonic agents. In the presence of normal renal function, these agents should produce an *(increase/ decrease)* in fluid excretion, or a *diuretic* effect.

out of

increase

13 *Note:* Both hypotonic and hypertonic solutions utilize the principles of *osmosis*. Another term for hypotonicity, then, is hyposmolarity.

Another term for hypertonicity, then, is _____.

hyperosmolarity

14 Solutions having the *same concentration* in relation to each other are *isotonic*. An isotonic solution administered into the body *(will/ will not)* alter the osmotic concentration. In this situation, movement of water *(would/would not)* occur. Examples of isotonic solutions are *normal saline* and *dextrose 5% in water.*

will not
would not

15 IN SUMMARY:

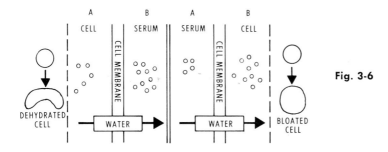

A
CELL

B
SERUM

A
SERUM

B
CELL

CELL MEMBRANE

CELL MEMBRANE

DEHYDRATED CELL

WATER

WATER

BLOATED CELL

Fig. 3-6

Homeostatic mechanisms

16 Many interacting forces in the body combine to maintain equilibrium, or _____. Osmosis is one of the processes by which fluid balance is regulated at the cellular level. Fluid and electrolyte balance is also regulated systemically via special areas in the body known as receptors.

homeostasis

17 Increases or decreases in intravascular fluid result in changes in blood *concentration* (tonicity or osmolarity).

Special areas in the body known as *osmoreceptors* are sensitive to changes in osmolarity, or _____.

concentration

18 Increases or decreases in body fluid also result in changes in blood volume, which may influence the *blood pressure*.
Special areas in the body known as *pressoreceptors* are sensitive to these changes in _____.

pressure

The pressoreceptors are located in the walls of the aortic arch, the internal carotid arteries, the juxtaglomerular apparatus in the kidneys, and the left atrium. They are sensitive to the *pressure* exerted on the vascular walls as they are stretched by the *volume* of blood leaving the heart—the *cardiac output.*

19 *Let us review:* Fluid and electrolyte balance is maintained systemically via receptor areas.
The osmoreceptors are sensitive to changes in _____.

concentration

The pressoreceptors are sensitive to changes in _____ _____.

cardiac output

The receptors control the secretion of hormones that regulate fluids and electrolytes in the kidney. The receptors thus act as mediators in the maintenance of fluid and electrolyte balance.

20 *Antidiuretic hormone* (ADH) is secreted by the posterior pituitary and inhibits excretion of water by the kidney, thereby causing water conservation. Secretion of ADH is stimulated by the osmolarity of extracellular fluid via the _____.

osmoreceptors

The *osmoreceptors* are located in a special area in the hypothalamus. These cells are bathed by the body's fluid. In the presence of hypotonicity, or *(increased/decreased)* osmolarity, the osmoreceptors *bloat* and in this way sense *(increased/decreased)* body fluid. In the presence of hypertonicity, or *(increased/decreased)* osmolarity, the osmoreceptors shrink and in this way sense *(increased/decreased)* body fluid.

decreased
increased
increased
decreased

So: Inhibition of ADH secretion leads to *(diuresis/water reabsorption)*.

diuresis

Increased ADH secretion leads to *(diuresis/water reabsorption)*.

water reabsorption

21

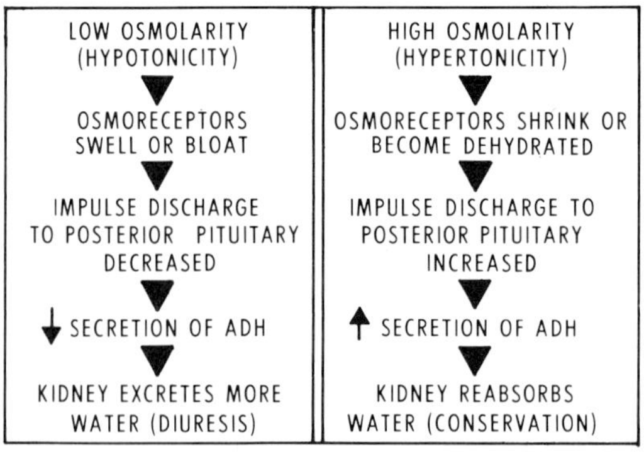

LOW OSMOLARITY (HYPOTONICITY)	HIGH OSMOLARITY (HYPERTONICITY)
▼	▼
OSMORECEPTORS SWELL OR BLOAT	OSMORECEPTORS SHRINK OR BECOME DEHYDRATED
▼	▼
IMPULSE DISCHARGE TO POSTERIOR PITUITARY DECREASED	IMPULSE DISCHARGE TO POSTERIOR PITUITARY INCREASED
▼	▼
↓ SECRETION OF ADH	↑ SECRETION OF ADH
▼	▼
KIDNEY EXCRETES MORE WATER (DIURESIS)	KIDNEY REABSORBS WATER (CONSERVATION)

Fig. 3-7

22 *Adrenoglomerulotropin* is a hormone released from an area of the diencephalon (inner brain) in response to a low cardiac output. Its release is thus mediated via the *(osmo-/presso-)* receptors. This hormone stimulates the adrenal cortex to produce aldosterone.

presso-

Therefore: Adrenoglomerulotropin stimulates the production of

_____.

aldosterone

23 *Aldosterone* is secreted by the adrenal cortex and causes the kidney to retain sodium ions (Na^+) and to excrete potassium ions (K^+).
Note: When Na^+ is retained, H_2O is also retained.
Secretion of aldosterone is stimulated by: adrenoglomerulotropin, angiotensin II, decreased Na^+ in the ECF, and increased K^+ in the ECF.

24 Another mechanism influencing the release of aldosterone is found in the kidney. The *renin-angiotensin mechanism* is stimulated when the juxtaglomerular apparatus in the kidneys senses decreased pressure and ischemia.
Renin is released secondary to pressure changes and acts as a catalyst in the synthesis of angiotensin II.
Angiotensin II causes vasoconstriction and aldosterone secretion.

Remember: Aldosterone causes Na^+ _____, water

_____, and K^+ _____.

reabsorption

*reabsorption;
excretion*

25 IN SUMMARY:

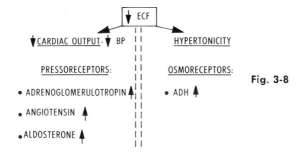

Fig. 3-8

26 The combined actions of the homeostatic mechanisms are shown in Figs. 3-9 and 3-10. As an example, we have considered the imbalance decreased *ECF volume.* We have illustrated the homeostatic responses to the two major problems presented with this imbalance: (1) ↓ *cardiac output* (reflected by a decreased blood pressure), and (2) ↑ *osmolarity* (seen as cellular dehydration).

27

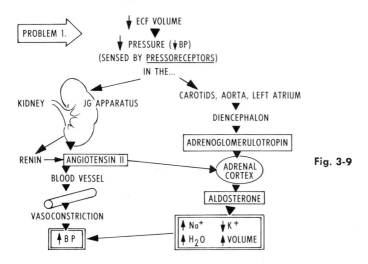

Fig. 3-9

28

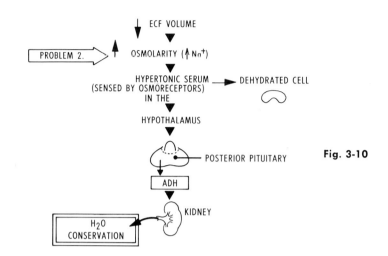

↓ ECF VOLUME

PROBLEM 2. ➔ ↑ OSMOLARITY (↑Na⁺)

HYPERTONIC SERUM ➔ DEHYDRATED CELL
(SENSED BY OSMORECEPTORS)
IN THE

HYPOTHALAMUS

POSTERIOR PITUITARY   **Fig. 3-10**

ADH

KIDNEY

H₂O
CONSERVATION

29 *So it can be seen that* the patient with decreased ECF volume may
present a clinical picture of *(increased/decreased)* blood pressure   *decreased*

and cellular _____, *and that* as the decreased ECF is cor-   *dehydration*
rected the secondary problems of *hypotension* and *cellular dehydra-*
tion will disappear.

30 Angiotensin II stimulates the secretion of the hormone

_____.   *aldosterone*
Angiotensin II therefore *(does/does not)* regulate fluid balance.   *does*
Angiotensin II also *(increases/decreases)* the blood pressure via   *increases*

the mechanism of _____.   *vasoconstriction*

The role of electrolytes in the conduction of electrical impulses

31 In the *polarized*, or resting, state, the inside of the cell is electrically *(negative/positive)* with respect to the outside. All of the   *negative*
body's "charged particles," or *ions*, contribute to the cell's charge.

32 Each ion is found both inside and outside of the cell. Therefore, Na⁺

and K⁺ are found both _____ and _____ of the cell.   *inside   outside*
K⁺ is found *primarily* inside the cell. Na⁺ is found *primarily*

_____ the cell.   *outside*

33 Every ion (Na⁺, Cl⁻, protein⁻) inside and outside the cell has its
own charge.
In the polarized, or resting, state the inside of the cell has a net negative charge. The inside of the cell is thus *(electronegative/electro-*   *electronegative*
positive) with respect to the outside.

34 Certain factors have been cited as contributing to the establish-
ment of this electronegativity. These factors are:
1. The presence of nondiffusable intracellular anions
Remember: Anions are *(positively/negatively)* charged particles.   *negatively*
2. The loss of intracellular potassium (a cation) as a result of enhanced membrane permeability

35 Let us now consider how impulses are conducted—the process of *de-*
polarization.
Remember: When depolarization occurs, the inside of the cell becomes electro*(positive/negative)* with respect to the outside.   *positive*

46

FACTORS CREATING THE
POLARIZED STATE

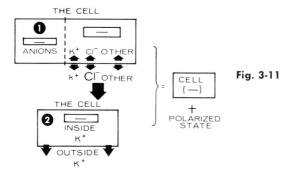

Fig. 3-11

37 *Sodium* plays a major role in the conduction of the impulse.
Remember: Sodium is a *(positively/negatively)* charged particle.   *positively*

38 It was mentioned earlier that some ions are found primarily inside
the cell, while others are found primarily outside the cell. Special
"gates" in the cell membrane limit the free diffusion of the ion particles so that a difference in intracellular and extracellular concentration of each ion is established.
Remember: The greatest concentration of Na^+ is found *(inside/out-*   *outside*
side) the cell.

39 When an electrical impulse reaches a resting cell membrane, the Na^+
gates open. Sodium ions rush *into* the cell, upsetting the previous
(electronegative/electropositive) relationship.   *electronegative*
Therefore, the cell loses its negativity and becomes *(electronegative/*
electropositive) with respect to the outside.   *electropositive*
The cell has then conducted the impulse and is said to be depolarized.

40 In order to receive another impulse, the cell must return to its previous resting, or _____, state. This stage is known as   *polarized*
_____.   *repolarization*

41 During this stage the cell closes its gates to sodium, thereby stop-
ping depolarization. The permeability of the cell membrane to K^+
increases as the cell "gates" of K^+ now open.
Remember: The greatest concentration of K^+ is found *(inside/out-*   *inside*
side) the cell.
Therefore, as the K^+ gates open, diffusion occurs, causing some of
the intracellular K^+ to move out of the cell. Because of this loss of
+ ions, the inside of the cell again becomes *(electropositive/electro-*   *electronegative*
negative) with respect to the outside, and the cell is said to have
been _____.   *repolarized*
Thus the major influence of K^+ is manifested during the *(depolar-*
ization/repolarization) phase of the cardiac cycle.   *repolarization*

42 The Na^+ that enters the cell during depolarization is returned to its
extracellular site in preparation for the next impulse via a pump exchange mechanism. The active pumping of Na^+ requires work, or
energy. The body's units of energy—ATP—are needed.
It is currently thought that the major role of the Na^+ pump is to

return the electrolytes to their original location. Its contribution to cell charge is thought to be negligible, since, for each Na⁺ ion pumped out of the cell, there is an equal replacement of a K⁺ ion back into the cell.

43 On the ECG, the QRS complex represents ventricular depolarization

and the T wave represents ventricular _____.
Na⁺ may be said to affect *(depolarization/repolarization)* and therefore the *(QRS/T wave)*.
K⁺ may be said to affect *(depolarization/repolarization)* and therefore the *(QRS/T wave)*.

44 An insult to the cell membrane (such as occurs in infarction) allows K⁺ to leak in and out of the cell freely, thereby disturbing electronegativity.

45 *Note:* Some have used these principles in formulating a mode of therapy in the management of acute myocardial infarction (MI). It has been theorized that if the electrical instability of infarction is affected by K⁺ instability, replacement of this K⁺ into the cell (in conjunction with glucose and insulin) should eliminate the electrical instability. Essentially, one creates his own K⁺ pump and cell membrane. This solution reportedly helps the injured cell to return to its previously polarized state. It is therefore known as a

_____ solution. Users claim fewer to no arrhythmias and   *polarizing*
accelerated healing. The use of polarizing solution in clinical practice, however, is still controversial.

46 IN SUMMARY:

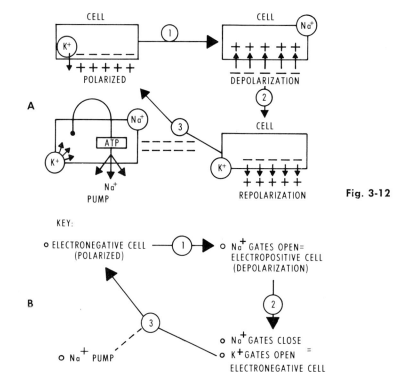

Fig. 3-12

48

47 Depolarization causes Ca^{++} to move into the cell, resulting in mechanical activity, or *contraction*.

Therefore, contractility is controlled by _____. Depolarization al- Ca^{++}
lows Ca^{++} to have its effect.

In this way, *electrical activity* and *mechanical activity* become related.

48 IN SUMMARY:

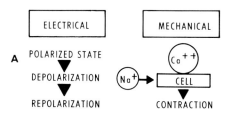

ECG CORRELATION:

Fig. 3-13

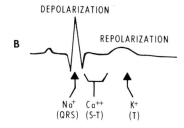

49 *Note:* The contractile effects of digitalis are related to its effect on
the calcium ion.

The action potential

50 In its resting, or polarized, state the cell has a potential for electrical activation—a *resting potential*. As the electronegativity of
the cell becomes greater, the resting potential also becomes greater.
Normal resting cell membrane potential is −90 mv.

51 When a single cell is activated by a stimulus, local electrical changes
occur producing an *action* current, or *action potential*.

This action potential from one cell can be recorded onto graphic
paper producing a pattern (Fig. 3-14).

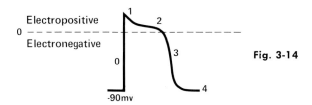

Fig. 3-14

52 The phase of electrical action denoted by **0** represents a change in

cellular polarity from electronegative to _____.   *electropositive*

Therefore, phase **0** represents the process of _____.   *depolarization*

53 The phase of electrical action denoted by **1, 2,** and **3** represent the

return to electronegativity, or _____.   *repolarization*

Phase 4 represents the resting membrane potential.

54 The action potential represents the electrical activity of (a) *(single/many)* cardiac cell(s).

single

A surface ECG represents the electrical activity of (a) *(single/many)* cardiac cell(s) recorded from the body surface.

many

The *surface* ECG, then, records the effects of (a) *(single/many)* action potential(s). As a result, only a rough correlation may be drawn between the events of cellular action potentials and the events of the surface ECG.

many

55 *Let us review:*

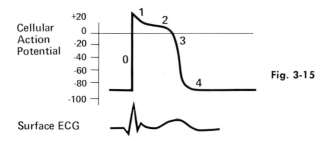

Fig. 3-15

Phase 0 of the action potential represents *(depolarization/repolarization)* in the single cardiac cell. Depolarization of many ventricular cells is reflected on the surface ECG as the _____ _____

depolarization

QRS complex

Therefore, the QRS complex reflects the phase ___ of many ventricular cells.

0

56 Phases 1, 2, and 3 of the action potential represent *(depolarization/repolarization)* in the single cardiac cell. Repolarization of many cardiac cells in the ventricles is reflected on the surface ECG by the

repolarization

_____ wave.

T

Note: The S-T segment correlates roughly to phases 1 and 2.

Fluid and electrolyte imbalances in the coronary care unit

57 The fluid and electrolyte imbalances most frequently seen in the setting of a coronary care unit are discussed in this section.

Fluid imbalances

58 Let us first consider the problem of *hypervolemia.*

Hypervolemia is a condition in which there is an excess of fluid volume in the *extracellular* fluid compartment.

Remember: The extracellular fluid consists of the _____

intravascular

fluid and the _____ fluid. Therefore, in a state of hyper-

interstitial

volemia, there is an excess of fluid between the _____ and also

cells

within the _____ _____. The excess of fluid between the cells results in *(intravascular/interstitial)* edema.

blood vessels
interstitial

59 The most common cause of hypervolemia in the setting of a coronary care unit is *congestive heart failure* (CHF).

In CHF the heart is weakened and cardiac output *(increases/decreases).*

decreases

This decrease in cardiac output results in a fall in blood pressure, which is sensed by the body's *(osmoreceptors/pressoreceptors).*

pressoreceptors

50

Remember: The pressoreceptors are sensitive to arterial stretch.

60 The pressoreceptors trigger a sequence of events, which causes an
increased production of the hormones _____ _____   *adrenoglomerulotropin*

and _____ _____. This stimulates the secretion of   *angiotensin II*

_____.   *aldosterone*
Aldosterone causes the reabsorption of _____ and the excretion of   *Na⁺*

_____ by the kidneys.   *K⁺*
Remember: When Na⁺ is reabsorbed, water is also retained.

61 Retention of Na⁺ and water by the kidneys leads to the development
of a state of *(hypervolemia/hypovolemia)*.   *hypervolemia*
In CHF, a state of hypervolemia imposes an increased strain on
an already weakened myocardium. Thus the compensatory mechanisms involved in this situation *potentiate* the underlying problem.

62 In this fluid imbalance, Na⁺ and water *(are/are not)* retained. How-   *are*
ever, more water than Na⁺ is usually retained. Thus the serum becomes *(hypotonic/hypertonic)*.   *hypotonic*
When the serum is hypotonic, the secretion of ADH would be ex-
pected to be *(increased/decreased)*. For some reason, however, the   *decreased*
fall in cardiac output associated with CHF paradoxically triggers
an *increased* secretion of ADH. Thus more fluid is retained, and
the compensatory mechanisms again potentiate the underlying
problem.

63 The clinical symptoms of hypervolemia associated with congestive
heart failure are: (1) interstitial and/or intracellular edema (peripheral, pulmonary); and (2) oliguria.

64 In the management of *hypervolemia* secondary to CHF, therapy is
directed toward: (1) decreasing cardiac workload through diuresis,
and (2) improving myocardial function.

65 *Let us review:* The most common cause of hypervolemia in the setting of coronary care is _____.   *CHF*
In the setting of CHF, there is a(n) *(increase/fall)* in cardiac out-   *fall*

put, which is sensed by the _____.   *pressoreceptors*
The pressoreceptors trigger a sequence of events, which causes a(n)

(increased/decreased) secretion of _____.   *increased; aldosterone*

Aldosterone causes reabsorption of _____ and _____ by the   *Na⁺   H₂O*

_____.   *kidneys*
The retention of Na⁺ and water results in *(hypovolemia/hypervole-*   *hypervolemia*
mia).
Diuretic agents *(may/may not)* be used in the management of hy-   *may*
pervolemia secondary to CHF.
Diuretics act to block the reabsorption of _____ and _____ by the   *Na⁺   H₂O*
kidneys.

66 Let us now discuss the problem of *hypovolemia*.
Hypovolemia is a condition in which there is a deficit of fluid in the
extracellular fluid compartment.
A common cause of hypovolemia in the setting of a coronary care
unit is excessive diuresis.

67 With excessive diuresis there is a(n) *(decrease/increase)* in blood volume and therefore a fall in cardiac output. — *decrease*

This fall in cardiac output is sensed by the *(pressoreceptors/osmoreceptors)*. — *pressoreceptors*

The pressoreceptors trigger an increased production of _____ and _____ _____, which — *adrenoglomerulotropin; angiotensin II*

then stimulate the secretion of _____. — *aldosterone*

Remember: Aldosterone causes the retention of _____ and _____, — *Na⁺* Na^+ *H₂O* H_2O

which leads to a(n) *(increase/decrease)* in blood volume. — *increase*

In this setting, the compensatory mechanisms are working toward

correcting the underlying problem of _____. — *hypovolemia*

68 With excessive diuresis, both _____ and _____ are excreted. However, more water than Na⁺ is usually lost, and the serum becomes *(hypertonic/hypotonic)*. — Na^+ H_2O — *hypertonic*

Remember: A hypertonic serum causes water to move *(into/out of)* the cells. This results in *(bloated/dehydrated)* cells. — *out of* — *dehydrated*

69 This hypertonicity is sensed by the *(osmoreceptors/pressoreceptors)*. This causes a(n) *(increase/decrease)* in the secretion of ADH. Thus water is *(conserved/excreted)*. — *osmoreceptors* — *increase* — *conserved*

Therefore, following excessive diuresis, the serum becomes *(hypotonic/hypertonic)*, the cardiac output *(increases/falls)*, and there is — *hypertonic* *falls*

cellular _____. — *dehydration*

70 The clinical symptoms of hypovolemia associated with excessive diuresis are dehydration, hypotension, and oliguria.

The management of this type of clinical problem is directed toward supporting the body's own homeostatic efforts by the administration of fluids.

	HYPERVOLEMIA	HYPOVOLEMIA
CLINICAL EXAMPLE	CHF	EXCESSIVE DIURESIS
SERUM	HYPOTONIC	HYPERTONIC
CELL	BLOATED	DEHYDRATED
SYMPTOMS	EDEMA OLIGURIA	DEHYDRATION HYPOTENSION OLIGURIA
THERAPY	DECREASE CARDIAC WORK LOAD IMPROVE CARDIAC FUNCTION	FLUID ADMINISTRATION

Fig. 3-16

Electrolyte imbalances

71 The electrolyte imbalances, particularly imbalances of *potassium* and *calcium,* frequently seen in the setting of a coronary care unit are discussed in this section.

72 Let us first consider the potassium imbalance known as *hypokalemia,* or low serum potassium levels.

The most common cause of hypokalemia in the coronary care unit is excessive diuresis.

73 Hypokalemia increases electrical instability by influencing the *polarized state*. Potassium is necessary for the maintenance of a stable polarized state. Therefore, hypokalemia may *(enhance/depress)* electrical instability, or automaticity, and cause ventricular arrhythmias.

enhance

74 *Remember:* Potassium affects the *(depolarization/repolarization)* phase of the cardiac cycle. Hypokalemia therefore affects the *(QRS/ T wave)* on the ECG.

repolarization

T wave

In the presence of hypokalemia repolarization is prolonged. There is *flattening* of the T wave and the appearance of an extra wave known as the *U* wave. The T wave and the U wave may fuse into one wave. This is known as the T-U _____ and is an electrocardiographic sign of _____.

fusion

hypokalemia

75 ECG evidence of *hypokalemia:*

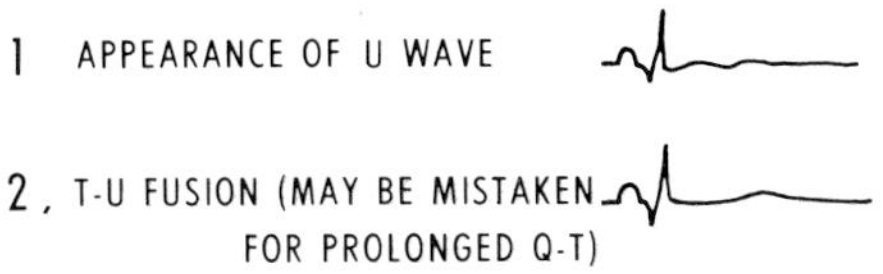

1   APPEARANCE OF U WAVE

2 . T-U FUSION (MAY BE MISTAKEN   **Fig. 3-17**
FOR PROLONGED Q-T)

76 The most common cause of hypokalemia is excessive _____.

diuresis

The management of hypokalemia is directed toward the replacement of the needed potassium via oral or intravenous supplements.

77 Other manifestations of hypokalemia are weakness and muscle cramps.

78 IN SUMMARY:

↓ K⁺ (HYPOKALEMIA)

BODY	● WEAKNESS ● MUSCLE CRAMPS
HEART	● ↑ ELECTRICAL INSTABILITY (↑ AUTOMATICITY) ● ⟶ VENTRICULAR ARRHYTHMIAS
ECG	● APPEARANCE OF U WAVE ● T-U FUSION
TREATMENT	● REPLACEMENT OF K VIA IV OR PO

Fig. 3-18

79 Let us now consider the problem of *hyperkalemia,* or high serum potassium levels.

The most common cause of hyperkalemia is failure to discontinue potassium supplements after diuresis.

80 *Remember:* Potassium affects the *(depolarization/repolarization)* phase of the cardiac cycle, or the ____ wave.

repolarization

T

Unlike hypokalemia, hyperkalemia is an electrical *(stimulant/depressant)*.

depressant

The cells repolarize quickly, although not effectively, since they do not become as electronegative as they are normally.

In comparison: if hypokalemia causes flattening of the T wave, then hyperkalemia should produce *peaking* of the ____ wave.

T

The earliest electrocardiographic sign of hyperkalemia is peaking

of the _____ wave. Peaking of the T wave is best visualized in the   *T*
midchest leads.

Note: The peaked T waves seen in hyperkalemia are symmetrical.

81 When repolarization is disturbed, the phase of *depolarization* may also become depressed. The next electrocardiographic sign of hyperkalemia is *widening* of the QRS complex.

82 The last sign of hyperkalemia on the ECG is disappearance of the P wave.

83 ECG evidence of *hyperkalemia:*

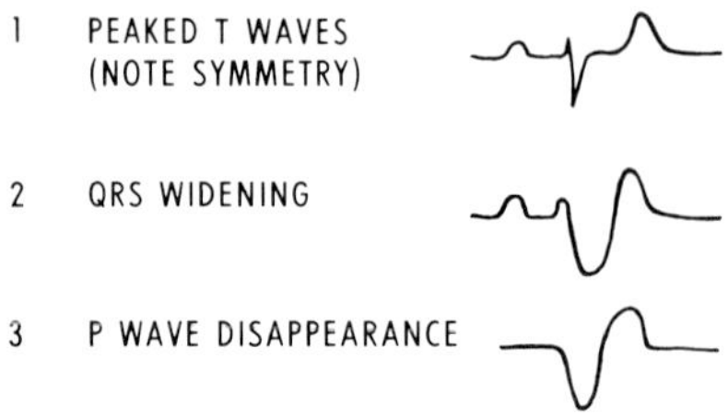

1   PEAKED T WAVES
(NOTE SYMMETRY)

2   QRS WIDENING   **Fig. 3-19**

3   P WAVE DISAPPEARANCE

84 It is important for nurses to be able to recognize the electrocardiographic manifestations of hyperkalemia *because immediate* treatment is indicated to correct the *cardiac depression* and *ventricular arrhythmias,* and to prevent *asystole.*

85 The management of hyperkalemia may be complicated if the imbalance is not detected in the early stages. In the terminal stage, the complexes *appear* wide and ventricular. They may be erroneously treated by a cardiac depressant, thereby potentiating the *(depressant/stimulant)* effects of the high potassium level.   *depressant*

86 The other manifestations of hyperkalemia are similar to those accompanying hypokalemic states:

1. _____   *weakness*

2. muscle _____   *cramps*

Note: It is difficult to distinguish potassium imbalances by clinical symptoms alone. Serum values and ECG evidence provide more information.

87 The management of hyperkalemia consists of:

ACUTE SITUATION	• Na HCO$_3$(SODIUM BICARBONATE)
	• GLUCOSE AND INSULIN
	• Ca^{++}
CHRONIC SITUATION	• ION EXCHANGE RESINS (KAYEXALATE)
	• DIALYSIS

Fig. 3-20

88 Na$^+$ and Ca^{++} may be given as cardiac *(stimulants/depressants).*   *stimulants*

Their effects counteract the _____ effect of the high potassium level.   *depressant*

The effects of hyperkalemia are caused by the *(serum/intracellular)*   *serum*
K$^+$. Glucose and insulin are given to push the excess K$^+$ *(into/out of)*   *into*
the cells of the body away from the heart. The sodium bicarbonate

produces an alkalosis, which *also* mobilizes K$^+$ *(into/out of)* the cells.

into

89 IN SUMMARY:

		$\downarrow$K$^+$ HYPOKALEMIA	$\uparrow$K$^+$ HYPERKALEMIA

BODY		o WEAKNESS
		o MUSCLE
		   CRAMPS
			o WEAKNESS
			o MUSCLE
			   CRAMPS

HEART		o$\uparrow$ ELECTRICAL
		   INSTABILITY
		   (AUTOMATICITY)
		o VENTRICULAR
		   ARRHYTHMIAS
			o CARDIAC
			   DEPRESSION
			o ASYSTOLE
			o VENTRICULAR
			   ARRHYTHMIAS

ECG		o APPEARANCE OF
		   U WAVE
		o T-U FUSION
			o PEAKED T WAVE
			o QRS WIDENING
			o DISAPPEARANCE
			   OF P WAVE

Fig. 3-21

90 Let us now consider the *calcium* imbalances.
The most common cause of calcium imbalances is an underlying acid-base imbalance.

91 *Hypocalcemia* refers to *low serum calcium* values.
Remember: The main role of Ca^{++} is in *contractility*.
Hypocalcemia will cause *(increased/decreased)* contractility of the heart. In the body, the opposite effect is seen—spasticity.

decreased

92 Ca^{++} has its effect between depolarization and repolarization.

Ca^{++} therefore affects the _____ segment on the ECG.
Hypocalcemia causes prolongation of the S-T segment, but does *not* affect the QRS complex or the T wave.

S-T

93 *Hypercalcemia* refers to a condition of high serum calcium values.
The most common cause of hypercalcemia is an underlying problem of *acidosis*.
Hypercalcemia will cause *(increased/decreased)* contractility of the heart. In the body, hypercalcemia causes the opposite effect—flaccidity.

increased

94 Hypercalcemia causes *(prolongation/shortening)* of the S-T segment and *(does/does not)* affect the QRS complex or the T wave.
Note: Calcium and digitalis act on the same portion of the cardiac cycle. Both are cardiac *(stimulants/depressants)* and affect the

_____ segment on the ECG.

shortening
does not

stimulants

S-T

95 Therapy in the management of calcium imbalances is usually directed toward correcting the underlying cause.

96 IN SUMMARY:

	$\uparrow$Ca^{++} HYPERCALCEMIA	$\downarrow$Ca^{++} HYPOCALCEMIA
BODY	FLACCID EXTREMITIES	SPASTIC EXTREMITIES
HEART	$\uparrow$ CONTRACTILITY	$\downarrow$ CONTRACTILITY
ECG	SHORTENED S-T SEGMENT	PROLONGED S-T SEGMENT

Fig. 3-22

ACID-BASE BALANCE
Definitions

97 An *acid* is a proton (H⁺) donor.

In the equation $H_2CO_3 \rightarrow (H^+) + HCO_3^-$ a hydrogen ion is given up;

therefore, the acid is _____. H_2CO_3

Note: H_2CO_3 is called carbonic acid.

A *base* is a proton (H⁺) acceptor.

In the same equation $H_2CO_3 \rightarrow (H^+) + HCO_3^-$ a hydrogen ion is ac-

cepted; therefore, the base is _____. HCO_3^-

Note: HCO_3^- is called bicarbonate and is usually bound with $Na^+ \rightarrow$ $NaHCO_3$.

98 Carbonic acid and bicarbonate are the most important of the body's acids and bases.

H_2CO_3 is a(n) *(acid/base)*. *acid*

HCO_3^- is a(n) *(acid/base)*. *base*

99 *pH* is the hydrogen ion concentration of the serum. Carbonic acid and bicarbonate occur in the body in a ratio of 20 to 1:

$$\frac{20 \text{ bicarbonates}}{1 \text{ carbonic acid}}$$

This ratio reflects the hydrogen ion concentration, or the _____. *pH*

Decreased pH = increased hydrogen ion concentration.

Increased pH = *(increased/decreased)* hydrogen ion concentration. *decreased*

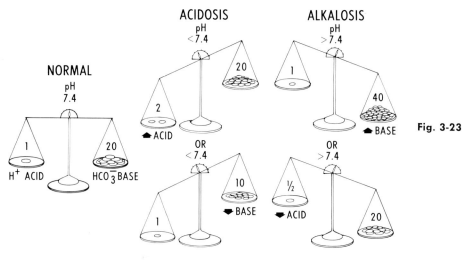

Fig. 3-23

100 *Acidosis* is a state of increased acid or decreased base.

A *low pH* corresponds to a *high hydrogen ion concentration* rela-

tive to the amount of base, which indicates _____. *acidosis*

Alkalosis is a state of increased base or decreased acid.

A *high pH* corresponds to a *low hydrogen ion concentration* rela-

tive to the amount of base, which indicates _____. *alkalosis*

The normal pH of arterial blood is 7.35 to 7.45.

A pH of 7.2 indicates _____. *acidosis*

A pH of 7.6 indicates _____. *alkalosis*

101 IN SUMMARY:

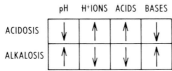

Fig. 3-24

	pH	H⁺IONS	ACIDS	BASES
ACIDOSIS	↓	↑	↑	↓
ALKALOSIS	↑	↓	↓	↑

102 Let us discuss the problem of *acidosis*.
Remember: Acidosis = a state of increased acid or decreased base.

103 There are two main sources of normal acid in the body:
1. cellular metabolism (work of the cells)
2. respiration (regulation of CO_2)

104 Acid may accumulate when there is abnormal _____ or *metabolism*

abnormal _____.   *respiration*
Note: Acid may also accumulate when there is abnormal excretion
of normally produced acids.
The end products of metabolism are excreted by the _____.   *kidneys*

The end products of respiration are excreted by the _____.   *lungs*

105 Acids may accumulate when there is *abnormal respiration*.

Lungs regulate acid-base balance by controlling levels of _____. CO_2
CO_2 can be converted to carbonic acid in the body: $CO_2 + H_2O \rightarrow$
H_2CO_3.
CO_2, then, can be considered an *acidic* substance. The lungs therefore regulate acid-base balance by controlling levels of *(acid/base)*.   *acid*

106 The level of CO_2 is controlled by *respiratory rate* and *depth*.
If a person breathes slowly or ineffectually, CO_2 will be *(retained/   retained
lost)*.
So: patients who retain CO_2 have *(increased/decreased)* levels of   *increased*

acid. This state is known as _____.   *acidosis*

107 Acid may also accumulate when there is *abnormal metabolism*.
When acid accumulates as a result of increased or abnormal cellu-

lar metabolism, a state of _____ results. When this occurs,   *acidosis*
the kidneys attempt to retain a substance that will balance out the
acidic effect.

108 A substance that balances an acid is a _____. The kidneys there-   *base*

fore regulate acid-base balance by regulating levels of _____.   *base*
Remember the equation: $H_2CO_3 \rightarrow (H^+) + HCO_3^-$

The body's most important base is _____. HCO_3^-
Therefore: to compensate for the increased acid, the kidneys re-

tain increased amounts of _____. HCO_3^-

109 Acid may also accumulate when normal acids are not excreted.
Remember: Acids are normally produced in the body. If these acids

are not excreted, a state of _____ will develop. One normal   *acidosis*

route of excretion of acids is the _____. Therefore: failure   *kidneys*

to excrete acids via the kidneys may lead to _____.   *acidosis*

110 IN SUMMARY: Acid may accumulate secondary to *metabolic* or *respiratory* causes.

Therefore: A patient can develop a _____ acidosis or a   *metabolic*

_____ acidosis.   *respiratory*

This relationship can be illustrated in a combined equation:

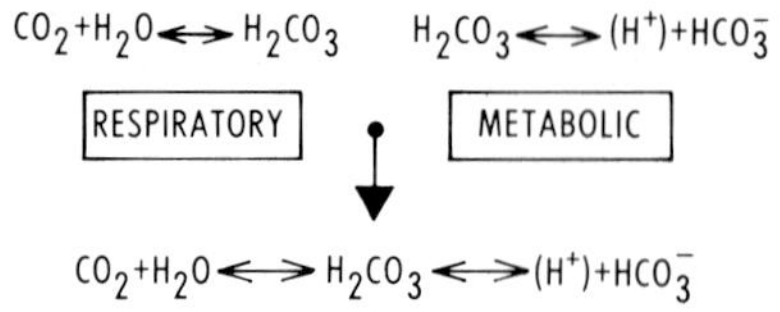

$$CO_2 + H_2O \longleftrightarrow H_2CO_3 \qquad H_2CO_3 \longleftrightarrow (H^+) + HCO_3^-$$

| RESPIRATORY | | METABOLIC |

Fig. 3-25

$$CO_2 + H_2O \longleftrightarrow H_2CO_3 \longleftrightarrow (H^+) + HCO_3^-$$

111 Let us discuss the problem of *alkalosis*.
Remember: Alkalosis is a state of increased base or decreased acid.

112 The kidneys *(can/cannot)* regulate base, or bicarbonate.   *can*

When the kidneys retain base, an _____ develops.   *alkalosis*
The lungs *(can/cannot)* directly regulate base, or bicarbonate.   *cannot*
The lungs *(can/cannot)* regulate acid, or CO_2.   *can*

113 If alkalosis is increased base or decreased acid, then the lungs create an alkalosis by *(losing acid/retaining base)*.   *losing acid*

Lungs lose acid in the form of _____. Therefore, alkalosis can be CO_2
caused by *(increased/decreased)* CO_2.   *decreased*
If respirations are increased, CO_2 will *(increase/decrease)*, and   *decrease*
the patient becomes *(acidotic/alkalotic)*.   *alkalotic*

114 IN SUMMARY: Acid may be lost secondary to respiratory causes.
Base may be retained secondary to metabolic causes.

Therefore: A patient can develop a _____ alkalosis or a   *respiratory*

_____ alkalosis.   *metabolic*

Metabolic acidosis

115 Metabolic acidosis results from increased levels of _____. The   *acid*
acid is usually a product of *abnormal metabolism*. However, metabolic acidosis can also result from decreased levels of base as may occur with excess loss from the lower GI tract due to diarrhea.
Note: Normal cell metabolism implies the glucose is metabolized in the presence of *oxygen*.

116 Some of the conditions that result in metabolic acidosis are diabetes, shock, and renal failure.
In *diabetes*, fats are metabolized for energy because there is not sufficient insulin available to metabolize glucose. The breakdown of fats releases acidic substances known as ketones. Diabetic aci-

dosis, therefore, is a _____ acidosis.   *keto-*
In *shock*, metabolism takes place without oxygen. This *anaerobic* metabolism results in the accumulation of lactic acid. The acidosis associated with shock is a _____ acidosis.   *lactic*
In *renal failure*, there is no abnormal metabolism, but the acidic products of normal metabolism may not be excreted. In renal failure the normal acids of metabolism are not excreted by the

_____.   *kidneys*

117 The clinical signs of metabolic acidosis are deep, rapid respirations and sensorium changes.

The lungs may assist the kidneys in the excretion of acids.
This is known as a *compensatory effort* of the lungs. The respiratory system compensates for a metabolic acidosis by excreting

acid in the form of _____. These patients will have *(increased/decreased)* respiratory rate and depth; for an example, consider the Kussmaul respirations seen in diabetic ketoacidosis.
Acidic substances are toxic to the tissues of the central nervous

CO_2 *increased*

system. The patient may also show _____ _____ secondary to this toxicity.

sensorium changes

118 In metabolic acidosis, the values obtained from arterial blood samples would be:
1. *(increased/decreased)* pH
2. *(increased/decreased)* HCO_3^-
In any acidosis, the pH is *(increased/decreased)*. In metabolic acidosis the kidneys and lungs are unable to keep up with the increased acid, and the bicarbonate value is *(increased/decreased)*.

decreased
decreased
decreased

decreased

Metabolic alkalosis

119 Metabolic alkalosis results from increased levels of _____ and/or loss of acid. Bicarbonate (HCO_3^-), a base, is reabsorbed in conditions in which chlorides (Cl^-) are lost from the body.
Principle: The body is always striving for homeostasis. When an anion (for example Cl^-) is lost, the body retains another anion (HCO_3^-) to compensate and to maintain the *(positive/negative)* charge.

base

negative

120 When Cl^- is lost, HCO_3^- is retained to maintain the body's *(negative/positive)* charge. However, bicarbonate can alter the acid-base balance of the body. When the body retains increased levels of

negative

bicarbonate or base, a state of _____ may develop.

alkalosis

121 Conditions that cause a loss of Cl^- from the body are diuresis, excessive vomiting, and gastrointestinal suction.
Note: These conditions also cause loss of acid.

122 *Remember:* In excessive diuresis, both water and K^+ are lost. Chlorides are lost with the K^+, so retention of _____ occurs. There-

HCO_3^-

fore, a _____ _____ can result.
In excessive *vomiting,* or *gastrointestinal suction,* HCl will be lost,

metabolic alkalosis

_____ will be saved, and a _____ _____ may result.

HCO_3^-; *metabolic alkalosis*

123 The clinical signs of metabolic alkalosis are slow, shallow respirations and symptoms of decreased Ca^{++} effect.
The lungs can help to compensate for the levels of increased base

by retaining _____ in the form of _____. By depressing and slowing respirations, CO_2 will be *(retained/lost)*.

acid CO_2
retained

124 *Remember:* Ca^{++} occurs in two forms: *free* (serum) and *bound* (to protein). The systemic effects of Ca^{++} are related to the levels of

free, or _____, Ca^{++}. Bound Ca^{++} may be considered to be *inactive* Ca^{++} because it is in a *stored* form. Alkalosis causes increased binding of Ca^{++} and a decrease in the levels of *(free/bound)* Ca^{++},

serum

free

thereby *(increasing/decreasing)* the effects of Ca⁺⁺. Therefore,   *decreasing*
the nurse can expect to see symptoms of *(hypocalcemia/hypercal-*   *hypocalcemia*
cemia) in the presence of alkalosis.

125 In metabolic alkalosis, the values obtained from arterial blood
samples would show:
1. *(increased/decreased)* pH   *increased*
2. *(increased/decreased)* HCO_3^- *increased*
In any alkalosis, the pH is *(increased/decreased)*. In metabolic al-   *increased*
kalosis the imbalance is caused by *(increased/decreased)* levels of   *increased*
base and/or *(increased/decreased)* levels of acid.   *decreased*

126 IN SUMMARY:

Fig. 3-26

Respiratory acidosis

127 Acidosis occurs when there are increased levels of *(acid/base)* or   *acid*
decreased levels of *(acid/base)*.   *base*

128 *Remember:* The lungs *(can/cannot)* directly regulate base or   *cannot*
HCO_3^-. But the lungs *(can/cannot)* regulate acid, in the form of   *can*

_____. CO_2
Respiratory acidosis is caused by *(increased/decreased)* levels of   *increased*
CO_2. The CO_2 is retained when the respiratory rate and depth are
(increased/decreased).   *decreased*

129 Some of the conditions that cause decreased or ineffective respirations are emphysema, drug overdoses (CNS depressants), and severe pulmonary congestion resulting from end stage acute respiratory failure.

130 In *emphysema*, patients are prone to the development of

_____ acidosis. The alveoli are damaged and CO_2 excretion   *respiratory*

is impaired. The subsequent retention of _____ may result in an CO_2
(alkalosis/acidosis). In *drug overdoses*, the respiratory center   *acidosis*
in the medulla may be depressed, resulting in *(increased/de-*   *decreased*

creased) respiratory rate and depth and the retention of _____. CO_2

131 Clinical signs of respiratory acidosis are decreased rate and depth
of respirations, and sensorium changes.
In respiratory acidosis, the respirations are *(increased/decreased)*.   *decreased*
The patient's respirations are the primary *cause* of the imbalance,

rather than acting as a _____ effort.   *compensatory*
The patient may also experience sensorium changes because
(acidic/alkaline) substances are toxic to the central nervous sys-   *acidic*
tem.

132 In respiratory acidosis, the arterial values are:
1. *(increased/decreased)* pH   *decreased*
2. *(increased/decreased)* P_{CO_2} *increased*
Remember: HCO_3^- is not considered when evaluating respiratory
imbalances.

Respiratory alkalosis

133 Alkalosis is a state of increased _____ or decreased _____.

base   *acid*

134 *Remember:* Respiratory acidosis is caused by *(increased/decreased)* respirations. Therefore, respiratory alkalosis would be caused by *(increased/decreased)* respirations.

decreased

increased

In the lungs, acid occurs in the form of _____. In respiratory alkalosis, the CO_2 levels are lowered by *(increasing/decreasing)* the

CO_2

increasing

respiratory rate and depth. The patient then "blows-off" _____.
Decreased levels of CO_2 create a state of decreased *(acid/base)*, or

CO_2

acid

_____.

alkalosis

135 Increased respiratory rate and depth can result from anxiety such as is manifested by a patient who is "fighting" a respirator. Anxiety causes a(n) *(increase/decrease)* in respirations and *(increased/decreased)* CO_2.

increase

decreased

136 An increase in respiratory rate also occurs in response to hypoxia in pulmonary edema. In early pulmonary edema CO_2 excretion may continue in the absence of effective O_2 transport because CO_2 diffuses more easily than O_2.

An increased respiratory rate causes *(increased/decreased)* CO_2 excretion. Therefore, in early pulmonary edema respiratory *(acidosis/alkalosis)* may be seen.

increased

alkalosis

137 The clinical signs of respiratory alkalosis are deep, rapid respirations, and symptoms of decreased Ca^{++} effect.

The deep, rapid respirations are the *cause* of the imbalance.

Alkalosis causes an increase in bound Ca^{++} and a(n) *(increase/decrease)* in free, or serum, Ca^{++}. This will result in symptoms of *(hypocalcemia/hypercalcemia)*.

decrease

hypocalcemia

138 The arterial blood gas values would be:
1. *(increased/decreased)* pH
2. *(increased/decreased)* P_{CO_2}

increased

decreased

139 IN SUMMARY:

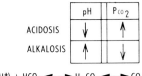

Fig. 3-27

$$(H^+) + HCO_3 \longleftrightarrow H_2CO_3 \longleftrightarrow CO_2 + H_2O$$

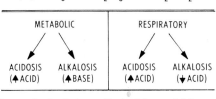

Fig. 3-28

140 *Note:* The three electrolytes affected by acid-base imbalances are: K^+, Ca^{++}, and Cl^-. The serum levels of these electrolytes will all appear *low* in a state of alkalosis. In contrast, serum levels of K^+,

Ca^{++}, and Cl^- are all *high* in a state of _____. The total body levels of K^+ and Ca^{++} may be normal, but their *location* may be altered. Potassium may move from the *intracellular* to *extracellular* fluid, and calcium may change from a state of *free* to *bound*.

acidosis

141 IN SUMMARY: Fill in the chart in Fig. 3-29 to indicate *increased* or *decreased* levels.

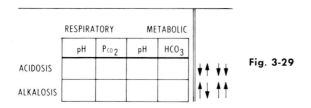

Fig. 3-29

Practical applications—arterial blood gases

142 Let us first consider the values that have been assigned to arterial blood gas levels by some institutions.

pH	7.35-7.45
Pco_2	35-45 mm Hg
HCO_3	22-26 mEq/liter

Note: These levels apply to a normal adult who is breathing room air. The values may vary in different institutional settings.

143 When analyzing a set of blood gas values, follow these steps:

Step 1—Check the pH: Is the value above or below normal? The pH value will indicate whether the problem is *acidosis* or *alkalosis.*

Note: Decreased pH = acidosis; increased pH = alkalosis.

Step 2—Check the values that reflect the *respiratory* side of the equation: Is the Pco_2 normal or increased or decreased?

Step 3—Check the value that reflects the *metabolic* side of the equation: Is HCO_3^- normal or increased or decreased?

144 The values may be applied in Fig. 3-30. Thus it can be further determined whether the problem is *metabolic* or *respiratory.*

	RESPIRATORY		METABOLIC	
	pH	Pco_2	pH	HCO_3
ACIDOSIS	↓	↑	↓	↓
ALKALOSIS	↑	↓	↑	↑

Fig. 3-30

145 Step 4—Make a diagnosis based on the fact that the pH will most likely indicate the primary disorder.

Step 5—Determine whether any compensatory mechanisms are involved; check the other values for abnormalities.

Step 6—Evaluate *why* the patient's blood gas values are abnormal, and decide the *medical* and *nursing action* to be taken.

146 Now apply the following values to a set of arterial blood gases.

pH 7.6
Pco_2 18 mm Hg
HCO_3^- 16 mEq/liter

147 According to the data given in frame 146:

The pH is *(increased/decreased/normal).*   *increased*

The pH indicates a(n) _____.   *alkalosis*
The Pco_2 value is *(increased/decreased/normal).*   *decreased*

62

The PCO_2 value indicates respiratory *(acidosis/alkalosis)*.

The $H\bar{C}O_3^-$ level is *(increased/decreased/normal)*.

The level of HCO_3^- indicates metabolic *(acidosis/alkalosis)*.

The pH indicates that the *primary* disorder is most likely

_____ _____.

The other changes most likely reflect the body's attempts at

_____.

148 Examples of conditions that might result in respiratory alkalosis include:
1. hyperventilation caused by anxiety
2. hyperventilation caused by hypoxia
Therapy is directed toward correction of the underlying mechanism.

Oxygenation: Po₂ and O₂ saturation

149 Two other values routinely obtained on a blood gas analysis are the PO_2 and O_2 saturation.
Analysis of the PO_2 and O_2 saturation allows us to evaluate the oxygen content of the blood. Oxygen is carried within the blood in two forms: (1) dissolved in solution and (2) bound to hemoglobin in the red blood cell for storage. The PO_2 reflects the pressure exerted by the amount of oxygen in solution. The O_2 saturation reflects the amount of oxygen bound to hemoglobin.

150 The bulk of the oxygen is carried in the storage form. Therefore, the greatest amount of information about the oxygen content available to the tissues is obtained from the *(PO_2/O_2 saturation)*.
Note: An O_2 saturation value of 97% or greater is fully acceptable as normal. Accuracy of O_2 saturation as a clue to O_2 content, however, is also dependent on the total hemoglobin content of the blood.

O_2 saturation

151 The PO_2 is useful in evaluating oxygen transport in the lungs. However, oxygen transport cannot be effectively evaluated without information about the amount of oxygen being delivered to the lungs. The percentage of oxygen being delivered to the patient is known as the F_1O_2 or fractional concentration of inspired oxygen. Delivery of an F_1O_2 of 1.0 is equivalent to delivering 100% oxygen.

152 Delivery of 100% oxygen across normal alveolar-capillary units results in the transport of enough oxygen into solution to exert a pressure of approximately 500 mm Hg (at sea level).
With delivery of 100% oxygen, then, the normal PO_2 should be approximately _____ mm Hg.

500

153 Delivery of 21% oxygen (room air) across a normal alveolar-capillary unit results in the transport of enough oxygen into solution to exert a pressure of approximately 100 mm Hg (at sea level).
With delivery of 21% oxygen, then, the normal PO_2 should be approximately _____ mm Hg.

100

Note: The normal PO_2 expected with adequate O_2 transport is about five times the F_1O_2 (at sea level):

F_1O_2 1.0 (100%) = PO_2 approx. 500 mm Hg
F_1O_2 0.2 (20%) = PO_2 approx. 100 mm Hg

F_1O_2 0.4 (40%) = Po_2 approx. _____ mm Hg

Variations in the expected Po_2 at a given F_1O_2 occur after the age of 60.

200

154 The state in which there is a lowered oxygen content in the *blood* is known as *hypoxemia*. The state in which there is insufficient oxygen at the *tissue* level is known as *hypoxia*.

155 The Po_2 and O_2 saturation allow us to evaluate oxygen content *(in the blood/at the tissue level)*. Therefore, changes in Po_2 and oxygen saturation may indicate *(hypoxia/hypoxemia)*.

in the blood
hypoxemia

Remember: Significant tissue hypoxia will result in metabolic changes leading to *(acidosis/alkalosis)*, which may be detected from the pH and bicarbonate values.

acidosis

156 IN SUMMARY: Lowered O_2 content of the blood is known as

_____.

hypoxemia

Hypoxemia is detected on a blood gas analysis by evaluating the

_____ and _____ _____.

Po_2   O_2 saturation

To determine if the lowered O_2 content is the result of interference in O_2 transport in the lungs, the Po_2 may be evaluated relative to the _____.

F_1O_2

Confirmation of associated tissue hypoxia is made by analyzing the

pH and _____ level.

bicarbonate

157 Tissue *utilization* of oxygen (O_2 consumption) is dependent on three major factors:
1. Changes in the metabolic demands (increased needs)
2. Changes in the cardiac output (increased or decreased amount of blood)
3. The O_2 content (increased or decreased O_2 content)

O_2 consumption = CO × O_2 content removed

158 Now apply all this new information to this set of arterial blood gas values.

pH	7.20
Pco_2	60 mm Hg
HCO_3^-	18 mEq/liter
Po_2	50 mm Hg
O_2 sat.	70%
F_1O_2	approx. 0.6 (60%): manual resuscitator (i.e. Ambu) approx. 15 liter/minute

159 According to the data given in frame 142:
The pH is *(increased/decreased/normal)*.

decreased

The pH indicates a(n) _____.
The Pco_2 level is *(increased/decreased/normal)*.
The Pco_2 indicates respiratory *(acidosis/alkalosis)*.
The HCO_3^- level is *(increased/decreased/normal)*.
The HCO_3^- indicates metabolic *(acidosis/alkalosis)*.

acidosis
increased
acidosis
decreased
acidosis

160 These arterial blood gases then indicate a combined _____

respiratory

and _____ acidosis and _____.

metabolic; hypoxia

An example of a condition that might result in such a picture is cardiorespiratory arrest.

161 The P_{O_2} and O_2 saturation values indicate that the oxygen content of the *(blood/tissues)* is *(decreased/normal)* and confirm, there- *blood; decreased*

fore, that a state of _____ exists. *hypoxemia*

Confirmation of associated *tissue hypoxia* is obtained from the pH

and the _____ level. *bicarbonate*

In the presence of an F_1O_2 of approximately 0.6 (60%) a P_{O_2} of

50 indicates *(normal/abnormal)* O_2 transport in the lungs. *abnormal*

162 Hypoxemia, hypoxia, and alteration in ventilation resulting in abnormal O_2 transport *(are/are not)* patient problems commonly oc- *are*
curring in cardiopulmonary arrest.
The therapy would be directed toward restoring more effective
ventilation, correcting the acidosis, and improving tissue oxygenation and perfusion.

Suggested readings

Baxter guide to fluid therapy, Morton Grove, Ill., 1969, Baxter Laboratories.

Beau, C. E., Braun, H., and Cheney, F.: Physiologic basis for respiratory care, Missoula, Montana, 1974, Mountain Press Publishing Co.

Beland, I. L.: Clinical nursing; pathophysiological and psychosocial approaches, New York, 1967, The Macmillan Co.

Broughton, J. O.: Understanding blood gases, Medical Director, Inhalation Therapy, Mercy Hospital, Denver, Colorado.

Castellanos, A., and Lemberg, L.: A programmed introduction to the electrical axis and action potential, Tampa Tracings, 1974.

Comroe, J.: Physiology of respiration, Chicago, 1971, Yearbook Medical Publishers, Inc.

Davenport, H. W.: The ABC of acid/base chemistry, Chicago, 1969, The University of Chicago Press.

Davis, J. O.: The mechanisms of salt and water retention in cardiac failure, Hosp. Pract., Oct., 1970.

Dubin, D.: Rapid interpretation of EKG's, Tampa, Fla., 1970, Cover Publishing Co.

Elek, S. R., and Laks, M. M.: Potassium and the electrocardiogram. In Bajusz, E., editor: Electrolytes and cardiovascular disease, Baltimore, 1966, The Williams & Wilkins Co.

Friedberg, C. K.: Diseases of the heart, Philadelphia, 1966, W. B. Saunders Co.

Ganong, W. F.: Review of medical physiology, Los Altos, Calif., 1969, Lange Medical Publications.

Guyton, A. C.: Textbook of medical physiology, Philadelphia, 1971, W. B. Saunders Co.

Hurst, W. J., and Logue, R. B., editors: The heart arteries and veins, New York, 1970, McGraw-Hill Book Co.

Lipman, B. S., Massie, E., and Klieger, R. E.: Clinical scalar electrocardiography, Chicago, 1972, Yearbook Medical Publishers, Inc.

Metheny, N. M., and Snively, W. D.: Nurses handbook of fluid balance, Philadelphia, 1967, J. B. Lippincott Co.

Netter, F. H.: Heart—The Ciba Collection of Medical Illustrations, Summit, N. J., 1967, Ciba Publications.

Netter, F.: Heart—The Ciba Collection of Medical Illustrations, Summit, N. J., 1969, Ciba Publications, pp. 48, 69.

Reed, G. M., and Sheppard, V. F.: Regulation of fluid and electrolyte balance; a programmed instruction in physiology for nurses, Philadelphia, 1971, W. B. Saunders Co.

Shapiro, B. A.: Clinical application of blood gases, Chicago, 1973, Yearbook Medical Publishers, Inc.

Soderman, W. A.: Pathologic physiology, ed. 4, Philadelphia, 1968, W. B. Saunders Co.

Sodi-Pallares, D., and others: Deductive and polyarametric electrocardiography, Mexico City, 1970, The National Institute of Cardiology.

Sodi-Pallares, D., and others: The polarizing treatment in cardiovascular conditions. In Bajusz, E., editor: Electrolytes and cardiovascular disease, Baltimore, 1966, The Williams & Wilkins Co.

Surawicz, B.: Evaluation of treatment of acute MI with potassium, glucose and insulin, Prog. Cardiov. Dis. 10:545, 1968.

Surawicz, B.: Relationship between electrocardiogram and electrolytes, Am. Heart J. 73(6): 814, June 1967.

The diagnosis of acute myocardial infarction

1 Myocardial infarction (MI) is death, or necrosis, of cardiac muscle resulting from an interrupted or diminished supply of oxygenated blood.
Acute myocardial infarction *usually* occurs as a result of a pathologic condition in the coronary artery system.
Remember: The heart receives its blood supply from two coronary

arteries, the _____ and the _____.   *right*   *left*

2 The majority of cases of acute coronary occlusion occur as a result of *atherosclerotic* heart disease. Atherosclerosis is characterized by thickening of the intima of the artery, which occurs as a result of fatty atheroma deposits, fibrosis, calcification, necrosis, and hemorrhage. These intimal changes lead to *narrowing*, or occlusion, of the coronary arteries.
Fig. 4-1 shows how atherosclerosis and thrombosis narrow the channel of the artery and decrease, or occlude, free flow of blood.

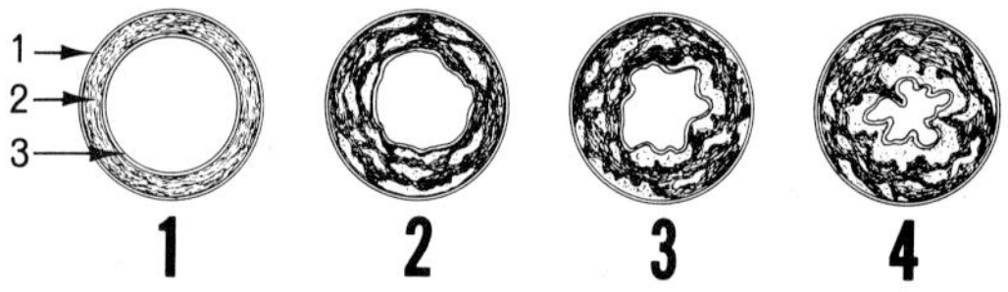

Fig. 4-1

1 2 3 4

3 Acute myocardial infarction is a clinical syndrome characterized by pain (which is usually *not* associated with exertion), left ventricular failure, signs of peripheral vascular collapse, fever, leukocytosis, and progressive electrocardiographic changes.
Another syndrome that results from a relative inadequacy of blood supply to the myocardium is known as *angina pectoris*. Angina pectoris is characterized by sudden attacks of retrosternal *pain* or oppression, which is triggered by exertion or other factors. The pain of angina pectoris is usually rapidly relieved by *rest* or by administration of *nitroglycerin*.

4 The diagnosis of acute myocardial infarction is based upon three interrelated components
1. history   2. serum enzymes   3. electrocardiographic changes

HISTORY

5 A "positive" history from a patient presenting with acute MI will usually include a description of characteristic *chest pain* and accompanying symptoms.
Pain is the presenting symptom in most patients with acute MI and will usually follow a characteristic pattern. Patients with acute MI may also *present* with signs of peripheral vascular collapse, nausea, and vomiting, diaphoresis, dyspnea and pulmonary congestion, and apprehension.

6 A complaint of chest pain must be assessed within the clinical setting in which it occurs. Chest pain may be caused by many different conditions, so it is important that other causes be ruled out. We will briefly consider three conditions in which the history may mimic acute myocardial infarction: angina pectoris, pericarditis, and pulmonary embolus.

7 See p. 68, Table 5.

8 *Nursing orders:* Chest pain
Remember: A "positive" history from a patient presenting with acute MI will usually include a description of characteristic *chest pain.*
1. Evaluate chest pain according to:
   — location
   — quality
   — duration
   — its association with respiration and change of position
   — accompanying symptoms—shortness of breath, dizziness, cold clammy skin, and nausea and/or vomiting
   — precipitating factors and mode of relief
2. Obtain vital signs and note any alterations in
   — blood pressure
   — pulse rate
   — respiratory rate
   Note: An increase in blood pressure is an expected response to pain. Wait until the pain is relieved and take blood pressure again.
3. Obtain a sample ECG tracing in the *inferior, lateral,* and *anteroseptal* monitoring leads. Analyze the ECG tracing and report for:
   — arrhythmias R wave
   — displacement of the S-T segment or changes in the T waves
   — abnormalities in the QRS morphology
   — changes in the polarity of the QRS complex
4. Relief of pain is a priority for any cardiac patient:
   — medicate promptly
   — record mode of relief: rest, nitroglycerin, morphine
5. Report immediately any chest pain that is:
   — different from that which has occurred before
   — accompanied by different symptoms
   — accompanied by changes in the ECG or vital signs
   — increasing in frequency and/or severity

SERUM ENZYMES

9 Enzymes are proteins that act as regulators of the chemical and metabolic activity of the *cells.* Therefore, enzymes are located *(inside/outside)* the cells.   *inside*

In the presence of cellular membrane destruction, enzymes are released into the bloodstream and the serum enzyme levels will *(increase/decrease).*   *increase*

Therefore, an elevation in serum enzymes indicate cellular

_____ _____.   *membrane destruction*

10 Characteristic enzymes are present in different types of cells. The enzymes that are present in *cardiac* cells are: (1) creatinine phosphokinase (CPK), (2) serum glutamic oxalacetic transaminase

Table 5

Question	MI pain	Angina	Pericarditis	Pulmonary embolus
Where do you feel the pain? (location)	Retrosternal, but may radiate to back, neck, arm, and jaw	Same	Located over the precordial area and to the back; may also radiate to jaw and arms	Usually over lung fields, to the side and the back
What is the pain like? (quality)	Pressure, choking, burning, tightness, viselike, usually *severe*	Similar in description to MI	Sharp ache in the chest; not necessarily severe but annoying	Similar to pericarditis, except to the side and the back
How long did it last? (duration)	At least 30 minutes	Relief usually in 15 minutes or less	Continuous; may last for days	Continuous for hours
Did you have any nausea? Did you feel short of breath? Did you feel weak and/or dizzy? Did you have cold sweats? (accompanying symptoms)	*May have*: nausea, dyspnea, weakness, diaphoresis, and dizziness	Usually *not* accompanied by diaphoresis or nausea	Usually *not* accompanied by these symptoms	Accompanied by *acute* shortness of breath, tachycardia, and apprehension (most characteristic—bloody sputum)
Was the pain relieved when you took a deep breath? (effects of respirations)	Not affected by respirations		Increased pain on inspiration	Increased pain on inspiration
Did you feel better when you sat up? (change of position)	Not relieved by change in position	May be only slightly relieved by change in position	Pain decreased on sitting up and increased when on *left* side	Decreased on sitting up
Was the pain relieved by anything?	Usually requires narcotics for relief	Relieved by rest when associated with *exertion*; relieved by nitroglycerin	Continuous soreness usually relieved somewhat by ASA or Tylenol	May be relieved with narcotics

(SGOT), (3) lactic dehydrogenase (LDH), and (4) alpha-hydroxy-butyrate dehydrogenase (HBD).

Therefore, in the presence of cardiac necrosis, there will usually be elevations in the levels of serum enzymes: _____, _____, _____, and _____.

CPK   *SGOT*

LDH   *HBD*

Levels of these enzymes may become elevated in the presence of any myocardial injury. Myocardial infarction, countershock, cardiac massage, and cardiopulmonary bypass could all *(elevate/decrease)* these enzyme levels.

elevate

11 Elevation of a single enzyme is not an indication of myocardial infarction.

Remember: Each enzyme is also present in other body tissues. CPK is also found in the tissues of the brain and skeletal muscle. Increased serum CPK levels are highly *specific* when abnormalities in the _____ muscle and _____ are excluded. It is also a highly *sensitive* enzyme since even small amounts of myocardial injury will cause it to become elevated.

skeletal   *brain*

SGOT may be released from many tissue other than the heart. Therefore, SGOT levels are highly *nonspecific* and of limited value. Conditions that may elevate the serum SGOT are liver disease, shock, profound tachyarrhythmias, and pulmonary infarction. An elevation of serum LDH is not specific for myocardial infarction. It may be elevated in the same conditions as SGOT. Also, LDH is found in red blood cells and may be released with hemolysis.

Elevation of serum HBD appears to be more specific than LDH and _____ for myocardial _____.

SGOT   *infarction*

The two most *specific* enzymes for myocardial injury are _____ and _____.

CPK

HBD

12 Following myocardial infarction, the levels of serum enzymes seem to follow a characteristic pattern.

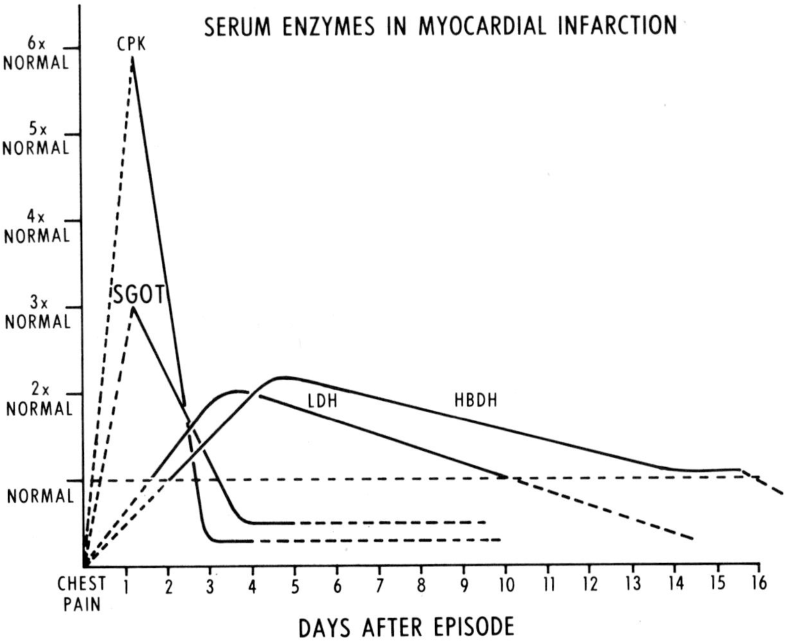

SERUM ENZYMES IN MYOCARDIAL INFARCTION

Fig. 4-2

DAYS AFTER EPISODE

13 It appears that the role of serum enzymes in the diagnosis of myocardial infarction is one of supporting the information gained from

the _____ and the _____.

history; electrocardiogram

14 Nurses should consider these points when serum enzymes are being evaluated:
   1. Avoid hemolysis of blood specimens.
       Remember: LDH is released from damaged _____ _____ cells.

red blood

   2. Note any intramuscular injections that are given or if an IV has been infiltrated.
       Remember: Enzymes may be released from injured skeletal

       _____.

muscle

   3. Note the use of countershock or cardiac massage that may

       increase serum enzyme levels and mimic _____

myocardial

       _____.

infarction

THE ELECTROCARDIOGRAM IN ACUTE MI

15 The ECG reflects the electrical activity of the heart as recorded on the body surface. Before discussing specific electrocardiographic manifestations of acute MI, let us consider the layers of the heart wall that are involved in myocardial infarction.

16 The wall of the heart is composed of three layers of ordinary muscle tissue.
    The layer of muscle tissue that lines the *interior* of the heart is

    known as the _____.

endocardium

    The *endocardium* is in direct contact with the blood pumped through the heart.
    The *outermost* layer of muscle tissue of the heart wall is known as

    the _____.

epicardium

    The endocardium has a poorer blood supply than the epicardium.
    Therefore, the endocardium is *(more/less)* vulnerable to any decrease in blood supply than is the epicardium.

more

    The layer of muscle tissue that lies *within* the endocardium and

    epicardium is known as the _____.

myocardium

    Remember: The epicardium is the *(outermost/innermost)* layer of tissue of the heart wall.

outermost

    Surrounding this layer is a membranous sac known as the pericardium.
    Between the epicardium and the pericardium is a potential space. A small amount of fluid is normally contained within this space and provides protection against mechanical friction.

17 A myocardial infarction may be limited to only one area of the heart wall.

ENDOCARDIUM   EPICARDIUM   Fig. 4-3

An infarction limited to the endocardium and the layer of muscle adjacent to the endocardium is known as a *subendocardial infarction.*

18 An infarction confined to the layer of muscle in the middle of the heart wall is known as an *intramural infarction.*

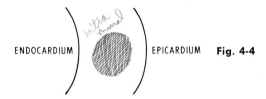

ENDOCARDIUM   EPICARDIUM   **Fig. 4-4**

19 An infarction limited to the layer of muscle below the epicardial tissue is known as a *subepicardial infarction.*

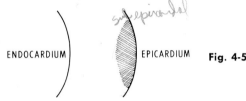

ENDOCARDIUM   EPICARDIUM   **Fig. 4-5**

20 The majority of infarctions are not limited to one area of the muscle but extend across the entire wall of the heart from the endocardium to the epicardium.

A myocardial infarction that *extends* from the *endocardium* to the *epicardium* is known as a *transmural* (across the wall) infarction.

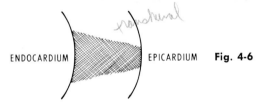

ENDOCARDIUM   EPICARDIUM   **Fig. 4-6**

Note: There is *always* more damage in the endocardial area than in the epicardial area in a transmural infarction.

Remember: The endocardium has a *(richer/poorer)* blood supply   *poorer*
than the epicardium and is therefore *(more/less)* vulnerable to a de-   *more*
crease in blood supply or oxygenation.

21 *Let us review:* An infarction limited to the layer of muscle below

the endocardium is known as a _____ infarction.   *subendocardial*
An infarction limited to the layer of muscle in the middle of the

heart wall is known as an _____ infarction.   *intramural*
An infarction that extends *across* the heart wall from the endocar-

dium to the epicardium is known as a _____ infarction.   *transmural*
The following discussion will focus on the *transmural* infarction, for it is the type most frequently diagnosed.

22 In this section the terms ischemia, injury, and necrosis are used to describe *electrical* events as seen on the ECG. These terms should not necessarily be equated with the physiologic phenomena they usually describe.

Remember: The term myocardial infarction means *physiologic death,* or necrosis, of cardiac muscle tissue. The electrical manifestation of necrosis, the abnormal Q wave, indicates that the cells are electrically dead but does not necessarily indicate that the cells are mechanically dead since documented abnormal Q waves are known to disappear.

Remember: The ECG is merely one of the parameters used in the clinically diagnosis of the myocardial infarction syndrome.

23 The earliest sign of myocardial infarction is the appearance of subendocardial ischemia and subendocardial injury. These early signs are usually rapidly masked by more significant changes and thus are often missed on the ECG.

24 The first stage in the electrocardiographic evolution of a transmural MI is *S-T segment elevation* in the leads reflecting the *injured epicardial* area. This is usually the first electrocardiographic manifestation of acute MI. In this stage, some of the injured cells may respond poorly to the activation process. As a result, there is also a decrease in the amplitude of the *R waves* in the leads overlying the *injured area.*

25 The next stage in the electrocardiographic evolution of an MI is the appearance of *abnormal Q waves.* Abnormal Q waves indicate electrical death, or the inability to transmit electrical impulses temporarily or permanently.

An abnormal Q wave is one that is wider than 0.02 second, is deeper than a fourth (¼) of the R wave, is associated with a loss in the amplitude of the R wave, and simultaneously appears in several leads (for example, in inferior wall infarction abnormal Q waves will appear in Leads II, III, and aVF).

Note: These criteria may be used only when evaluating Q waves in Leads I, aVF, and V_6.

In this stage, there is still evidence of myocardial injury. This is because a zone of injury always surrounds an area of necrosis.

26 The next stage is that of ischemia. Symmetrical *inversion* of the *T wave* denotes electrical ischemia. Ischemia is superimposed upon injury and necrosis. Therefore, in this stage, T wave inversion

will be seen in conjunction with _____ elevation and abnormal _____ waves.

S-T

Q

27 ECG changes in acute MI:

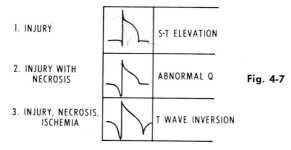

1. INJURY		S-T ELEVATION
2. INJURY WITH NECROSIS		ABNORMAL Q
3. INJURY, NECROSIS, ISCHEMIA		T WAVE INVERSION

Fig. 4-7

28 In the next stage, the current of injury subsides, but the necrosis and ischemia are still present.

Remember: Abnormal _____ waves denote myocardial necrosis.

Q

Symmetrical inversion of the _____ waves denotes myocardial _____.

T

ischemia

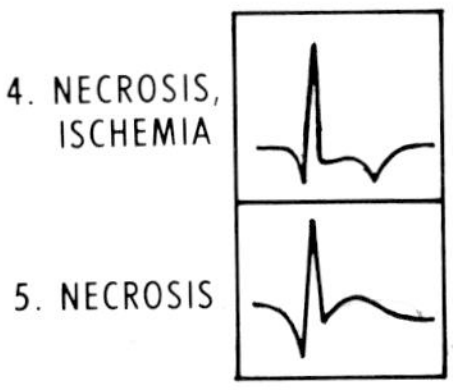

4. NECROSIS, ISCHEMIA

5. NECROSIS

Fig. 4-8

The ischemia may then subside. The only electrocardiographic manifestation of infarction which then remains is the abnormal _____ wave.

Q

29 In some patients, the abnormal Q wave may subsequently disappear. *Note:* The duration of each stage of infarction will vary from patient to patient.

30 The ECG changes described occur in the leads directly reflecting the area of infarction.
Indirect electrocardiographic evidence of *myocardial injury* may be obtained from the leads that are *opposite* the *injured area.*

31 *Remember:* Myocardial injury produces S-T segment _____ in the leads overlying the injured area. In the leads *opposite* the injured area, opposite, or *reciprocal,* changes will be seen. These changes are a *mirror* image of the ECG changes associated with the injury current.
Thus reciprocal changes are manifested on the ECG as S-T segment

elevation

(elevation/depression) in the leads directly _____ the injured area.
In the setting of acute MI, S-T segment elevation in the inferior

depression   *opposite*

leads will produce S-T segment _____ in the lateral leads.
S-T segment elevation in the lateral leads will produce S-T segment

depression

ment _____ in the inferior leads.

depression

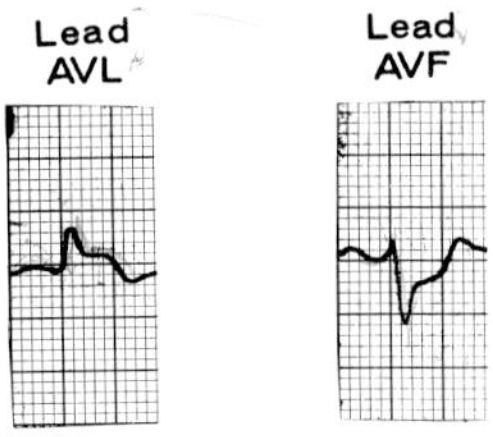

Lead AVL   Lead AVF

Fig. 4-9

32 *Let us review:* The stage of *ischemia* is characterized on the ECG by symmetrical abnormalities in the _____ waves.
The stage of *injury* is characterized by abnormal displacement of

T

the _____ segment.
The stage of *necrosis* is characterized by the appearance of *abnor-*

S-T

mal _____ waves.
The first electrocardiographic manifestation of acute MI is usually

Q

_____ _____ elevation in the leads overlying the injured area.

S-T segment

The appearance of abnormal Q waves indicates that there is an area

of electrical _____.   *necrosis*

Symmetrical *inversion* of the T wave denotes myocardial

_____.   *ischemia*

During the stage of injury, this disturbance in cellular metabolism is accompanied by *cell membrane damage.* Therefore the cells in the injured area are also *electrically unstable.* Ventricular arrhythmias may occur as a manifestation of this electrical instability. Because some of the cells in an area of injury may respond poorly to the activation process, there may also be decreased contractility in an injured area.

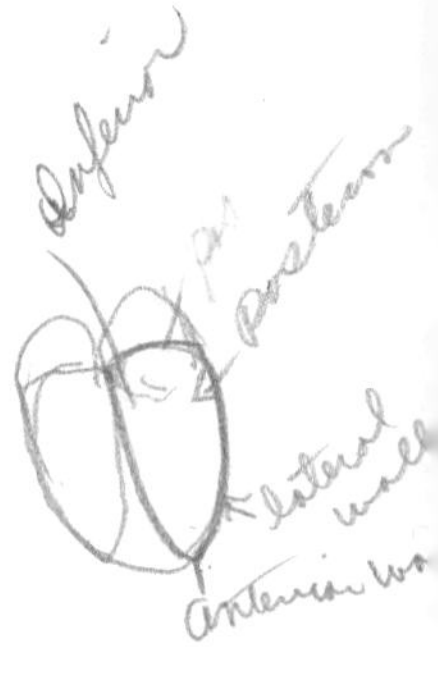

INFARCTION SITES

33 Knowledge of the anatomic location of an infarction enables us to anticipate the types of complications that are likely to occur. In this discussion, we will consider four surfaces of the *left ventricle:* (1) the anterior wall, (2) the lateral wall, (3) the inferior wall, and (4) the posterior wall.

34 *Remember:* The blood supply to the left ventricle is from both the

_____ and _____ coronary arteries.   *right   left*

Let us review: The *right* coronary artery primarily supplies the

(inferoposterior/anterolateral) surface of the left ventricle.   *inferoposterior*

The left coronary artery primarily supplies the *(inferoposterior/ anterolateral)* surface of the left ventricle. The left coronary artery has two main branches: *anterolateral*

1. the left anterior _____   *descending*

2. the left _____   *circumflex*

The anterior descending branch primarily supplies the _____   *anterior*

surface of the left ventricle.

The circumflex branch primarily supplies the _____ surface of   *lateral*

the left ventricle.

35 *Note:* When discussing acute myocardial infarction, it is important to consider the location of the occlusion in the coronary artery tree. Occlusions that occur high in the tree will produce more extensive damage than those in the smaller branches.

Extensive anterior wall myocardial infarction

36 Let us first consider infarctions that occur as a result of *left* coronary artery pathology.

Remember: The left coronary artery has two main branches. If an occlusion occurs in the *main* trunk of the left coronary artery, an infarction may occur in both the septal and lateral areas of the

_____ wall of the left ventricle.   *anterior*

EXTENSIVE ANTERIOR WALL MI:

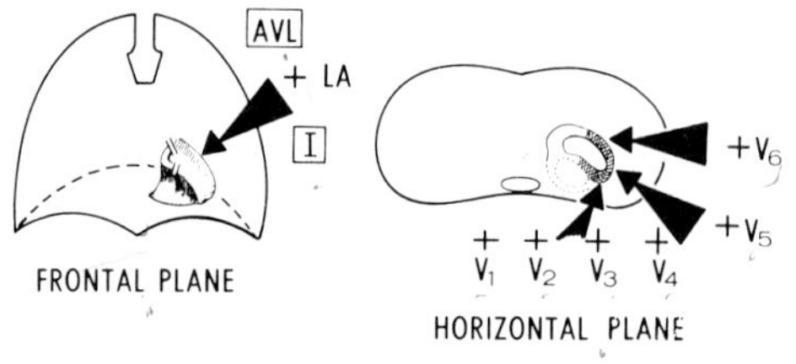

FRONTAL PLANE

HORIZONTAL PLANE

Fig. 4-10

37 The leads that reflect the electrical activity of the *septal* and *lateral*

areas of the left ventricle are Leads I and _____ and V_1 through   *aVL*

_____. Therefore, massive infarctions of the anterior wall may pro- V_6
duce changes in these leads.

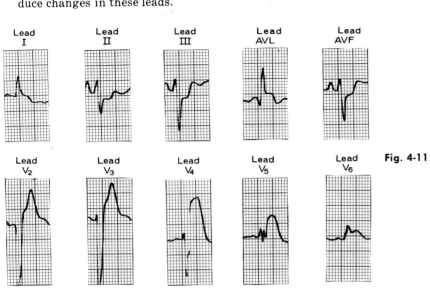

Fig. 4-11

Note: The S-T segment elevation in the V leads and Leads I and
aVL. The reciprocal changes are in the inferior leads.

Anteroseptal wall myocardial infarction

38 *Remember:* The left coronary artery has two main branches: the

left _____ _____ and the left _____.   *anterior descending;*
Occlusion of the left anterior descending branch will usually pro-   *circumflex*
duce infarction of the septal area of the anterior wall.
This is commonly referred to as anteroseptal wall MI.

ANTEROSEPTAL MI:

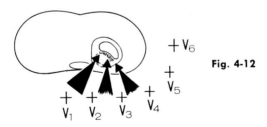

Fig. 4-12

HORIZONTAL PLANE

39 The leads that reflect the electrical activity of the anteroseptal wall

of the left ventricle are Leads V_1 through _____. Therefore, infarc- V_4
tions of the anteroseptal wall will produce changes in these leads.
Note: Leads V_2 and V_3 lie *directly* over the septum.

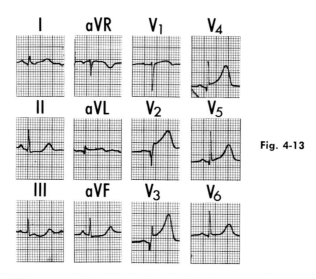

Fig. 4-13

Note: The S-T segment elevation in Leads V_1 through V_4.
There are no posterior positions on the six standard chest leads.
Therefore, reciprocal posterior wall changes reflecting anteroseptal
injury *(are/are not)* usually seen.   *are not*

Lateral wall myocardial infarction

40 Occlusion of the circumflex branch of the left coronary artery will
produce infarction of the lateral area of the anterior wall.

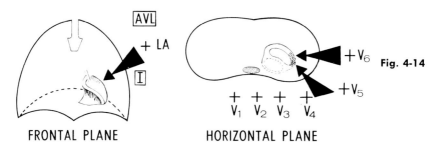

Fig. 4-14

41 *Remember:* The electrode that looks directly toward the lateral sur-

face of the left ventricle is the _____ arm electrode. The leads   *left*
that use the left arm electrode as their positive electrode are Leads

_____ and _____. Therefore, these leads are used in the diagnosis   *I*   *aVL*
of lateral wall MI. Leads V_4, V_5, and V_6 are *also* used when diagnosing lateral wall MI.

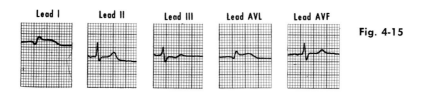

Fig. 4-15

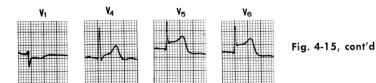

V_1 V_4 V_5 V_6

Fig. 4-15, cont'd

Note: The S-T segment elevation in Leads I, aVL, V_4, V_5, and V_6 and the reciprocal changes in the inferior leads.

42 In addition to supplying a *large* portion of the muscle mass of the left ventricle, the left coronary artery also supplies these structures:
1. the right bundle branch
2. the anterosuperior division of the left branch
3. the posteroinferior division of the left branch (a portion)
4. the anterior two-thirds of the ventricular septum
With this information, we can anticipate the types of problems that will occur as a result of left coronary artery pathology.

43 Left coronary occlusion commonly produces necrosis of large areas of left ventricular musculature. Therefore, it may be expected that patients with anterior wall MI will frequently present with *pump failure* more severe than that which accompanies right coronary artery pathology.
Therefore, patients with *left coronary artery* pathology are prone

to the development of _____ _____ and its accompanying arrhythmias.   *heart failure*
The arrhythmias that classically occur as a manifestation of heart failure are (1) sinus tachycardia and (2) rapid atrial arrhythmias.
Therefore, these arrhythmias are frequently seen in the presence of anterior wall MI.

44 It has also been stated that the left coronary artery supplies important structures of the *intraventricular* conduction system: the

right _____ _____, the antero-_____ division of the   *bundle branch; superior*

left branch, and a portion of the postero-_____ division of   *inferior*
the left branch. Therefore, it can be expected that intraventricular conduction disturbances will frequently accompany *left* coronary artery pathology. (See Unit 6.)
The arrhythmia that occurs as a result of blocks in the intraventricular conduction system is *Type II*, or *Mobitz, block.* (See Unit 5.)

45 *Let us review:* The left coronary artery has two main branches:

(1) the left _____ _____, and (2) the left   *anterior descending*

_____.   *circumflex*
Occlusion of the main trunk of the left coronary artery usually pro-

duces extensive _____ wall MI.   *anterior*
The leads used in the diagnosis of extensive anterior wall MI are

Leads _____ and _____ and _____ through _____.   *I   aVL V_1 V_6*
Occlusion of the anterior descending branch of the left coronary artery usually produces _____ wall MI. The leads used   *anteroseptal*

in the diagnosis of anteroseptal wall MI are _____ through _____.
Occlusion of the circumflex branch of the left coronary artery usu-

V_1 V_4

ally produces _____ wall MI. The leads that reflect the electri-

lateral

cal activity of the lateral wall are _____ and _____ and V_4, _____,

I   aVL V_5

and _____.

V_6

It can be expected that patients with left coronary artery occlusion

will frequently present with: (1) heart _____ and (2)

failure

_____ conduction disturbances.

intraventricular

46 *Nursing orders:* The patient with left coronary artery occlusion
1. Anticipate the development of heart failure.
   — check lungs for rales
   — auscultate heart for gallops
   — check fluid balance and CVP readings
   — *Remember:* the arrhythmias commonly associated with heart

   failure are sinus _____ and rapid _____ arrhyth-

   tachycardia   atrial

   mias
2. Monitor the patient for the development of intraventricular conduction disturbances and A-V blocks. (Type II Mobitz block and
   its precursors) (see Unit 6)

Inferoposterior wall myocardial infarction

47 Let us now consider infarctions that occur as a result of right coronary artery pathology.
Remember: The right coronary artery primarily supplies the *(an-
terolateral/inferoposterior)* wall of the left ventricle. Although it is

inferoposterior

relatively uncommon for *infarction* to extend across the entire inferoposterior wall, it is common for these two walls to be *injured*
simultaneously. Most frequently, infarction is limited to the inferior wall, and the injury current extends to the posterior wall. As
the infarction evolves the posterior wall injury often subsides.

INFERIOR-POSTERIOR WALL MI.

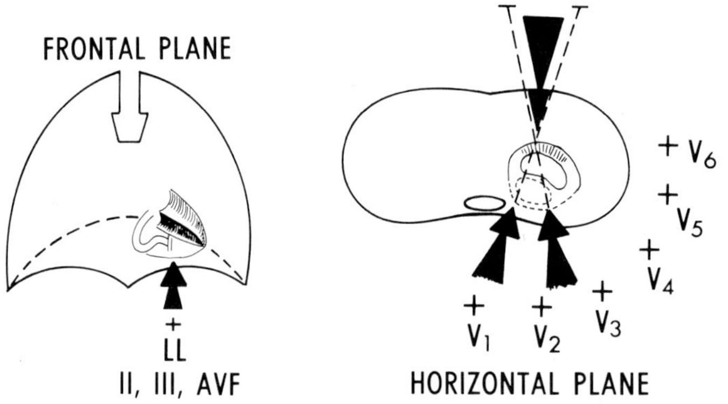

FRONTAL PLANE

LL
II, III, AVF

HORIZONTAL PLANE

$+V_6$
$+V_5$
$+V_4$
$+V_3$
$+V_1$ $+V_2$

Fig. 4-16

48 The foot electrode looks directly toward the inferior surface of the

_____ ventricle. The leads that use the foot electrode as their

left

positive electrode are _____, _____, and _____. Therefore, Leads

II   III   aVF

II, III, and aVF are used in the diagnosis of _____ wall MI.

inferior

There is no electrode that looks directly toward the posterior surface of the left ventricle. Therefore, in order to detect the electrical activity in the posterior wall we must consider the leads located directly opposite this area. Leads V_1 and V_2 are thus used in the diagnosis of _____ wall MI.

posterior

Remember: Injury is manifested by S-T segment *(elevation/depression)* in the leads reflecting the injured area. Therefore, in the leads opposite the injured area we would expect to see S-T segment

elevation

_____.

depression

49 Posterior wall injury is thus reflected in Leads V_1 and V_2 as S-T segment *(elevation/depression)*. Electrical death, or necrosis, is represented by an abnormal Q wave in the leads reflecting the area of necrosis. Therefore, in the leads opposite an area of necrosis we would expect to see *(Q waves/R waves)*. Thus in the presence of posterior wall necrosis there is an increase in the amplitude of the R waves in Leads _____ and _____.

depression

R waves

V_1 V_2

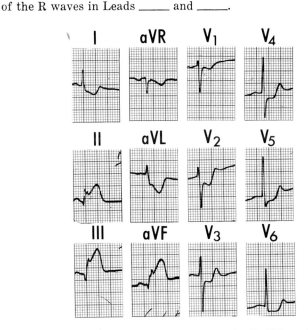

Fig. 4-17

Note: The S-T segment elevation in Leads II, III, and aVF and the S-T segment depression in V_1 and V_2.
Also, there are reciprocal changes in Leads I and aVL.

50 In addition to supplying the inferoposterior surface of the left ventricle, the right coronary artery usually also supplies these structures:
1. the _____ node

S-A

2. the _____ _____ tissue

A-V junctional

3. bundle of His
4. posterior one-third of the _____

septum

5. posteroinferior division of the _____ branch (a portion)

left

With this information, we can anticipate the types of problems that will occur as a result of right coronary artery pathology.

51 Right coronary artery occlusion commonly causes ischemia to the

S-A node, A-V junctional tissue, and the parasympathetic (vagal) fibers supplying these structures. As a result of this ischemia, *bradyarrhythmias,* or slow rates, occur. The specific bradyarrhythmias commonly associated with right coronary occlusion are: (1) sinus bradycardia and (2) Type I, or Wenckebach, block.

52 *Let us review:* The right coronary artery primarily supplies the *(inferior/anterior)* surface of the left ventricle.   *inferior*

Occlusion of the right coronary artery commonly produces   *inferior*

_____ wall MI.

The leads used in the diagnosis of inferior wall MI are Leads _____,   *II*

_____, and _____.   *III*   *aVF*

It can be expected that patients with right coronary artery occlusion will frequently present with *(bradyarrhythmias/tachyarrhythmias).*   *bradyarrhythmias*

53 *Nursing orders:* The patient with right coronary artery occlusion
1. Anticipate *bradyarrhythmias:*
   — sinus bradycardia
   — first-degree A-V block
   — Type I, or Wenckebach, second-degree A-V blocks
2. Watch for arrhythmias that may break through in the presence of slow rates (see Unit V)
3. Have *atropine* at the bedside
4. Be cautious in the administration of depressive drugs such as *morphine* or with vagal stimulation such as rectal temperatures

Posterior wall myocardial infarction

54 Let us now consider infarctions confined to the posterior wall of the left ventricle. Formerly, the terms *inferior* and *posterior* were used synonymously. Although they are frequently injured simultaneously, these two areas have now been identified as two *separate* surfaces of the left ventricle.

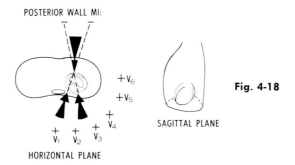

Fig. 4-18

The *inferior* surface of the left ventricle is that which rests against the diaphragm. The "true" *posterior* surface of the left ventricle is that which lies closer to the atria.

55 Infarctions limited to the "true" posterior wall of the left ventricle usually occur as a result of occlusion of the circumflex branch of the left coronary artery.

Infarctions of the posterior wall frequently occur in *conjunction* with infarctions of the inferior wall. Inferoposterior infarctions occur as a result of right coronary artery occlusions.

56 *Remember:* Leads V_1 and V_2 are used in the diagnosis of

_____ wall MI. In the presence of posterior wall MI, there is   *posterior*
an increase in the amplitude of the R waves in Leads V_1 and V_2.

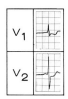

Fig. 4-19

PERICARDITIS

57 A more diffuse form of myocardial injury is that which occurs with
pericarditis.
Remember: The pericardium is a membranous _____ that surrounds   *sac*
the epicardium on the *(inside/outside)* of the heart. Inflammation   *outside*
of the pericardium is known as *pericarditis.*

58 The pericardium surrounds the entire heart. Inflammation of the
pericardium, therefore, produces a *(localized/diffuse)* injury.   *diffuse*
Inflammation produces pain. Inflammation of the pericardium produces *chest* pain. Therefore, the clinical picture of pericarditis
(may/may not) confuse the differential diagnosis of acute MI.   *may*

Both pericarditis and myocardial infarction produce _____ pain.   *chest*
Pericarditis differs from myocardial infarction, however, because
it represents a *(localized/diffuse)* myocardial injury.   *diffuse*

59 Pericarditis may not be related to coronary artery disease. However, it may occur in the setting of *myocardial infarction.* This is
because the injury extends to the epicardium and therefore easily

affects the _____.   *pericardium*

60 Myocardial injury is reflected on the ECG by ____ _____   *S-T segment*
elevation.

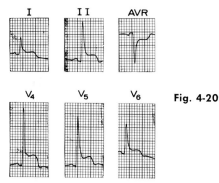

Fig. 4-20

Pericarditis produces *(localized/diffuse)* myocardial injury. The   *diffuse*
ECG changes produced will also be diffuse. In the presence of peri-
carditis, S-T segment elevation is seen in *all* the epicardial leads.
Reciprocal changes will be seen only in the endocardial lead, Lead

_____.   *aVR*
Note: When pericarditis is superimposed on myocardial infarc-

tion, the former reciprocal S-T depression associated with the infarction will either disappear or become elevated.

Suggested readings

Andreoli, K. G., and others: Comprehensive cardiac care, ed. 3, St. Louis, 1975, The C. V. Mosby Co.

Chapman, B. L.: Correlation of mortality rate and serum enzyme in myocardial infarction, Br. Heart J. 33:643-649, 1971.

Cohen, L.: Contributions of serum enzymes and isoenzymes to the diagnosis of myocardial injury, Mod. Concepts Cardiov. Dis. 26:49, 1967.

DePasquale, N. P.: The electrocardiogram in complicated acute myocardial infarction, Prog. Cardiov. Dis. 13:1, 1970.

Dixon, S. H., Jr., and others: Changes in serum creatinine phosphokinase activity following thoracic, cardiac, and abdominal operations, Arch. Surg. 103:66-88, 1971.

Dubin, D.: Rapid interpretation of EKG's, Tampa, Fla., 1970, Cover Publishing Co.

Edwards, J. E.: The value and limitations of necropsy studies in coronary artery diseases, Prog. Cardiov. Dis. 13:4, 1970.

Eliott, W. C., and Garlin, R.: The coronary circulation, myocardial ischemia, and angina pectoris, Mod. Concepts Cardiov. Dis. 35:111, 1966.

Friedberg, C. K.: Diseases of the heart, Philadelphia, 1966, W. B. Saunders Co.

Hurst, W. J., and Logue, B. R., editors: The heart arteries and veins, New York, 1970, McGraw-Hill Book Co.

James, T.: The coronary circulation and conduction system in acute MI, Prog. Cardiov. Dis. 11:410, 1968.

Mariott, H. T. L.: Practical electrocardiography, Baltimore, 1968, The Williams & Wilkins Co.

Michie, D. D., and others: Serum enzyme changes following cardiac catheterization with and without selective coronary arteriography, Am. J. Med. Sci. 260:11-20, July 1970.

Netter, F. H.: Heart—The Ciba Collection of Medical Illustrations, Summit, N. J., 1969, Ciba Publications.

Neutze, J. M., and others: Serum enzymes after cardiac surgery using cardiopulmonary bypass, Am. Heart J. 88(4):425, Oct. 1974.

Sampson, J. J., and Chetlin, M. D.: Pathophysiology and differential diagnosis of cardiac pain, Prog. Cardiov. Dis. 14:507, 1971.

Schamroth, L.: An introduction to electrocardiography, Edinburgh, 1971, Blackwell Scientific Publications.

Shell, W., Kjekshus, J. K., and Sobel, B.: Qualitative assessment of the extent of myocardial infarction in the conscious dog by means of analysis of serial changes in serum creatine phosphokinase activity, J. Clin. Invest. 50: 2613-2614, 1971.

Sobel, B., and Shell, W.: Serum enzyme determinations in the diagnosis and assessment of myocardial infarction, Circulation, XLV:471-479, Feb. 1972.

Sodi-Pallares, D., and others: Deductive and polyparametric electrocardiography, Mexico City, 1970, The National Institute of Cardiology.

Sprague, H. B.: Examination of the heart, New York, 1965, The American Heart Association.

Winsor, T.: The electrocardiogram in myocardial infarction, Summit, N. J., 1968, Ciba Publications.

Electrical complications in acute myocardial infarction—arrhythmias

1 The heart has been described as having both electrical and mechanical properties.

The *three* electrical properties of the heart are: (1) _____,   *automaticity*

(2) _____, and (3) _____.   *excitability;*
Remember: *conductivity*
The ability of the heart to *initiate electrical* impulses is known as

_____.   *automaticity*
The ability of the heart to *respond* to electrical impulses is known

as _____.   *excitability*
The ability of the heart to *transmit* electrical impulses is known as

_____.   *conductivity*

2 When there are disturbances in the electrical activity of the heart, arrhythmias occur.

Arrhythmias, then, are manifestations of abnormal _____   *electrical*

_____.   *activity*
Generally, arrhythmias may be considered to be a result of disturbances in *automaticity* or *conduction* or *both*.
Note: Arrhythmias are considered to be *ectopic* when they originate outside the SA node.
Before discussing the pathophysiology of arrhythmias, let us again consider the innervation of the heart and its relationship to *automaticity* and *conduction*.

3 The heart is richly innervated by both sympathetic and parasympathetic nerves.

Remember: The sympathetic nervous system supplies the _____   *S-A*

node, the _____ muscle, the _____ _____ tissue, and   *atrial; A-V junctional*

the _____ muscle.   *ventricular*
Sympathetic stimulation: (1) *(increases/decreases)* automaticity   *increases*
in the S-A node; (2) *(accelerates/slows)* A-V conduction. Para-   *accelerates*

sympathetic (vagal) fibers supply the _____ node, the _____   *S-A   atrial*

muscle, and the _____ _____ tissue.   *A-V junctional*
Parasympathetic stimulation: (1) *(increases/decreases)* automa-   *decreases*
ticity in the S-A node; (2) *(accelerates/slows)* A-V conduction.   *slows*
Thus the sympathetic and parasympathetic nervous systems

strongly influence the properties of _____ and   *automaticity*

_____.   *conduction*

PATHOPHYSIOLOGY OF ARRHYTHMIAS

4 Arrhythmias may be *generally* considered as resulting from distur-

bances in _____ and/or _____.
    automaticity;
    conduction

Automaticity is the ability of certain areas of the heart to

_____ electrical impulses. The areas of the heart that *normally*
    initiate

have the property of automaticity are the _____ node, the _____
    S-A   *A-V*

_____ tissue, and the _____ system in the
    junctional   *His-*
ventricles.
    Purkinje

In the presence of certain pathology, the atria can also have the
property of *automaticity.*

5 Enhanced automaticity may cause arrhythmias that arise from

these same areas: the _____ node, the _____, the _____
    S-A *atria* *A-V*

_____ tissue, or the _____ system in the
    junctional   *His-*
ventricles.
    Purkinje

Increased automaticity may result in tachyarrhythmias, or *(slow/*

fast) rates.
    fast

The tachyarrhythmias

6 Tachyarrhythmias are potentially clinically significant because they
may cause a symptomatic *fall* in *cardiac output*, increase the oxygen
demands of the myocardium, and decrease coronary blood supply.
Some factors that have been identified as enhancing automaticity in
acute MI are:
1. ischemia, as occurs in the zone surrounding infarction
2. stretch, as occurs in congestive heart failure
3. electrolyte imbalance (hypokalemia)
4. drugs such as digitalis, Isuprel, epinephrine, aminophylline
5. sympathetic stimulation
6. acidosis and alkalosis
7. stress

Let us review: Increased automaticity may result in tachyarrhyth-

mias, or _____ rates.
    fast

7 Normally, the sinus node fires at the fastest rate and is the

_____ of the heart.
    pacemaker

When automaticity is enhanced, the atria, A-V node, or the ventri-

cles may assume control of the X_____.
    rhythm

An electrolyte imbalance that causes increased automaticity and

thus results in arrhythmias is X_____.
    hypokalemia

Some drugs that have the potential for increasing automaticity in

acute myocardial infarction are _____, _____,
    digitalis   *Isuprel*

and _____.
    aminophylline

Stretching of the myocardial fibers, which occurs in CHF, can also

cause increased _____.
    automaticity

Increased automaticity results in *(tachyarrhythmias/bradyarrhyth-*
    tachyarrhythmias
mias).

Tachyarrhythmias become clinically significant *when* they cause

a symptomatic fall in _____ _____, increase the
    cardiac output

_____ _____ of the myocardium, or decrease the   *oxygen demands*

_____ _____ _____.   *coronary blood supply*

8 Disturbances in automaticity may be considered in terms of their effect on the electrical events of single cells.
Remember: When a single cell is activated by a stimulus, local electrical changes occur producing an *action current*, or *action potential*. This action potential from one cell can be recorded onto graphic paper producing a pattern. (See Chapter 3, Frames 50 to 56.)

The action potential represents the electrical activity of *(a single/*   *a single*
many) cardiac cell(s). The *surface* ECG records the effects of *(a*
single/many) action potential(s).   *many*

9 The myocardial cells at rest have the potential for electrical activation due to the effective maintenance of an electronegative state by the cell membrane. This potential is usually sustained until an electrical stimulus arrives.

10 Cells with unstable membranes are not able to sustain an electronegative state. They begin to lose their electronegativity prematurely and thus depolarize spontaneously.

Action Potentials from any Automatic Cell (Ex. SA Node)

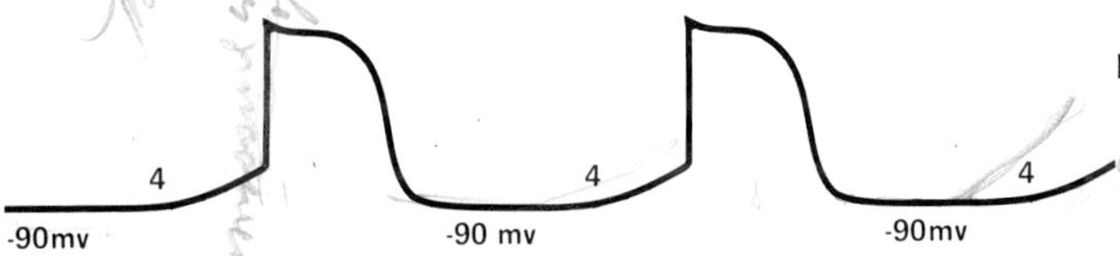

Fig. 5-1

-90mv   -90 mv   -90mv
     4   4   4

11 Automatic cells are electrically *(stable/unstable)*. They depolarize   *unstable*
spontaneously and prematurely—i.e., during electrical *diastole*, or phase 4.

Therefore, the property of automaticity is also referred to as phase

4 depolarization or spontaneous _____ depolarization.   *diastolic*

12 Automatic cells must reach a certain level of membrane potential before an action potential is generated. This level is known as the cell's *threshold potential.*

0 ——————

          B   B
     A   A

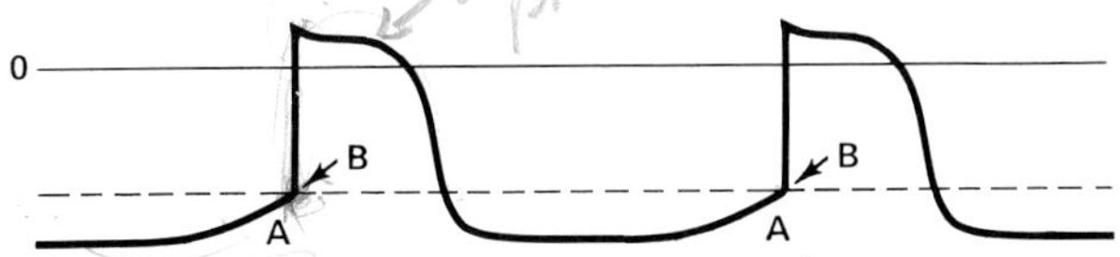

Fig. 5-2

The automatic cell in Fig. 5-2 begins to depolarize during the pe-

riod indicated by the letter _____. However, an *action potential* (ac-   *A*
tual impulse) is not generated until the time indicated by the letter

_____.   *B*

Therefore, this cell's *threshold potential* is denoted by the letter

_____.   *B*

Threshold potential is that level of membrane potential at which a

cell may generate an _____ _____.   *action potential*

13 Tachyarrhythmias are produced in the presence of enhanced

_____ (i.e., enhanced phase _____ depolarization).   *automaticity*   *4*
   Tachyarrhythmias may also be produced in the presence of *altered
   conduction.*

14 Altered conduction of a normal impulse may result in the genera-
   tion of an ectopic impulse. Altered conduction of normal impulses
   occurs when there has been asynchronous recovery or repolarization of previous impulses.

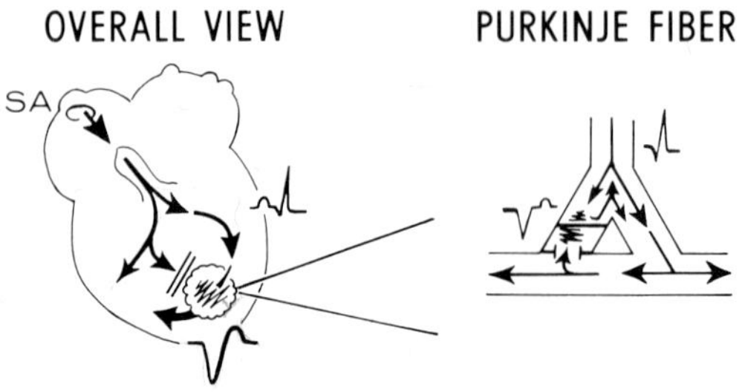

OVERALL VIEW   PURKINJE FIBER

Fig. 5-3

RE-ENTRY

15 When there is altered repolarization of an area of the heart, an impulse may be blocked from entering and being conducted evenly
   through this tissue. The impulse detours around the blocked en-
   trance area and travels through the abnormal tissue. When it exits,
   it re-enters and reactivates the heart. As the heart is reactivated,
   a new impulse is generated.
   This phenomenon, whereby an ectopic impulse is generated by the
   re-entry of a normal impulse into previously refractory tissue, is

   known as the _____ phenomenon.   *re-entry*

16 If an impulse is generated early in repolarization when the dispar-
   ity in recovery is especially pronounced, the impulse may continue
   to recycle in a circuit producing a chain reaction response.
   Remember: The period when a chain reaction response occurs is

   known as the _____ _____.   *vulnerable period*

17 Some factors that may enhance the occurrence of re-entry by altering repolarization are:
   1. ischemia
   2. electrolyte imbalance
   3. drugs
   4. acid-base imbalances
   5. surgical incisions (areas of edema)
   Note: These factors are very similar to those that enhance automaticity.

18 Since the formation of the re-entrant ectopic impulse is closely related to the preceding impulse, the ectopic beat occurs at a fixed distance from the beginning of the original impulse.
   This fixed distance is known as the *coupling interval.*

ECG SUPPORT:

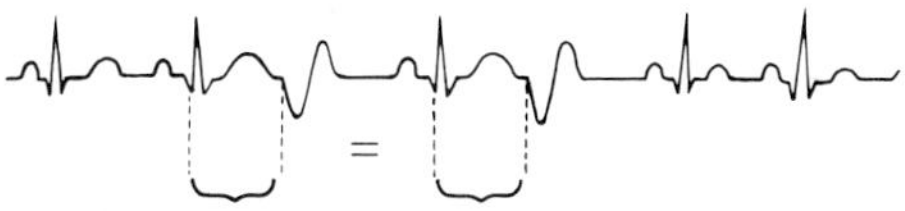

COUPLING INTERVALS

Fig. 5-4

When ectopic beats of the same focus occur at fixed coupling intervals, their mechanism of origin is *most likely (automaticity/re-entry)*.

re-entry

19 *Let us review:* Tachyarrhythmias are produced in the presence of

enhanced _____ or altered _____.

automaticity;
  conduction

Altered conduction of impulses may result in the formation of ectopic impulses by the mechanism of _____.

re-entry

The bradyarrhythmias

20 When automaticity and/or conduction are *depressed*, bradyarrhythmias, or *(fast/slow)* rates, occur.

slow

In the presence of depressed automaticity, the rate of impulse discharge from automatic centers *(decreases/increases)*.

decreases

When conduction is depressed, the transmission of an impulse may be delayed or blocked in any structure of the conduction system.

Depressed automaticity and depressed conduction often occur together and thus in conjunction cause bradyarrhythmias, or _____ rates.

slow

21 Bradyarrhythmias are potentially clinically significant because: (1) they may cause a symptomatic fall in cardiac output, and (2) they may allow for the breakthrough of dangerous tachyarrhythmias.

Some factors that have been identified as depressing automaticity and conduction are: (1) ischemia or infarction of the conduction structures, (2) electrolyte imbalance (hyperkalemia), (3) drugs such as digitalis, Inderal, quinidine, Pronestyl, and (4) parasympathetic stimulation to the vagal fibers (vagal stimulation) as occurs with ischemia.

22 *Let us review:* Depressed automaticity and depressed conduction

both cause bradyarrhythmias, or _____ rates.

slow

When automaticity is decreased, the rate of impulse discharge from

automatic centers _____. The areas of the heart that have

decreases

the property of automaticity are: the _____ node, the _____, the

S-A   atria

_____ _____ tissue, and the _____ system in the ventricles.

A-V junctional; His-
  Purkinje

When conduction is depressed or slowed, an impulse may be delayed

or _____ in any structure of the conduction system.

blocked

The electrolyte imbalance that depresses automaticity and conduction is _____.

hyperkalemia

Some drugs that have the ability to depress automaticity and con-

duction are: _____, _____, _____ and

digitalis; Inderal;
  quinidine

_____.

Pronestyl

Ischemia to the conduction structures or the _____ *parasympathetic*
nerve fibers can also depress automaticity or conduction.
Remember: Depressed automaticity and/or depressed conduction

cause _____ rates, or _____ arrhythmias. *slow   brady-*
Bradyarrhythmias are clinically significant *when* (1) they cause a

symptomatic fall in _____ _____, and when (2) they al- *cardiac output*

low for the breakthrough of _____ _____. *dangerous tachyar-*
rhythmias

IDENTIFICATION OF ARRHYTHMIAS ON THE ECG

23 When identifying arrhythmias, the following systematic approach
has been suggested.

1. Analyze the _____ complex. *QRS*

2. Analyze the _____ wave. *P*
3. Analyze the relationship between the P wave and the QRS

_____—the _____ interval. *complex   P-R*
The first part of the ECG to be considered is the _____ complex. *QRS*
Remember: The QRS complex represents depolarization of the

_____. *ventricles*

24 Analysis of the QRS complex provides information about the origin of the ventricular impulse. The origin of the impulse may be
ventricular or *supraventricular.*
If the impulse originates *in the ventricles,* the rhythm is described

as _____. *ventricular*
If the impulse originates *above the ventricles,* the rhythm is de-

scribed as _____. *supraventricular*

Remember: The structures above the ventricles that have the abil-

ity to initiate impulses are: the _____ node, the _____, and the *S-A   atria*

_____ _____ tissue. *A-V junctional*
Therefore sinus, atrial, and nodal or junctional arrhythmias are

classified as _____ arrhythmias. *supraventricular*
Supraventricular impulses are usually transmitted through the *nor-*
mal A-V conduction pathways to the ventricles.
When an impulse reaches the ventricles through these normal A-V
pathways, the ventricular musculature is depolarized *rapidly* and
the resulting QRS complex is *narrow.*
Thus supraventricular impulses will *usually* produce *(narrow/wide)* *narrow*
QRS complexes.
If we considered one patient, we would expect that *all* impulses aris-
ing *above* the ventricles should be conducted similarly through the
A-V node, His bundle, and bundle branches to reach the ventricles.
Therefore, all supraventricular impulses in a particular patient
should produce QRS complexes having the *same* configuration.
Supraventricular impulses may therefore be described as producing
QRS complexes that are *(narrow/wide)* and unchanging. *narrow*

25 Impulses arising in the ventricles *(are/are not)* transmitted through *are not*
the normal conduction pathways. As a result, depolarization of
the ventricular musculature occurs *slowly* or with *delay.* Thus ventricular impulses *usually* produce a QRS complex that is *(narrow/*
wide). Another characteristic of ventricular impulses is that they *wide*

88

will *always* produce QRS complexes different from the patient's normal complexes.

Ventricular impulses may therefore be described as producing QRS

complexes that are *usually (narrow/wide)* and *always* _____   *wide*   *different*
from the patient's normal complexes.

Thus, analysis of the QRS complexes enables us to ascertain

whether the origin of an impulse is _____ or   *ventricular*

_____.   *supraventricular*

26 Analysis of the P wave and calculation of the atrial rate aids in the differential diagnosis of supraventricular arrhythmias. Analysis of the P-R interval provides information about the relationship between the atria and the ventricles and aids in the diagnosis of atrioventricular (A-V) blocks.

Note: The origin of the rhythm is determined first. Next the discharge sequence—rate or timing of the impulse—is determined; and finally the conduction sequence is noted.

DISTURBANCES IN SINUS NODE FUNCTION

27 *Remember:* The sinus node normally has the property of *automaticity.*

Normally, electrical impulses arise from the sinus node and drive

the heart at a rate of _____ to _____ beats per minute.   *60   100*

Note: The sinus rate may be calculated on the ECG by measuring

the _____ wave rate. (See Unit 2.)   *P*

Sinus tachycardia

28 When automaticity in the sinus node is enhanced, impulse discharge
will *(increase/decrease)*.   *increase*

Increased automaticity in the sinus node may result in an arrhyth-

mia known as _____ tachycardia.   *sinus*

Sinus tachycardia generally falls in the range of *101* to *150* beats per minute.

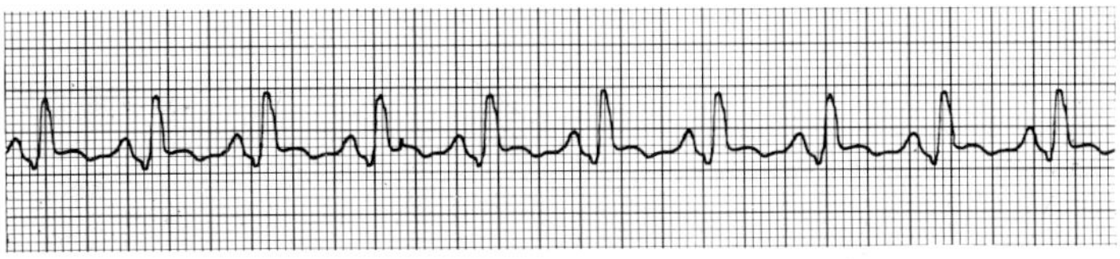

Fig. 5-5

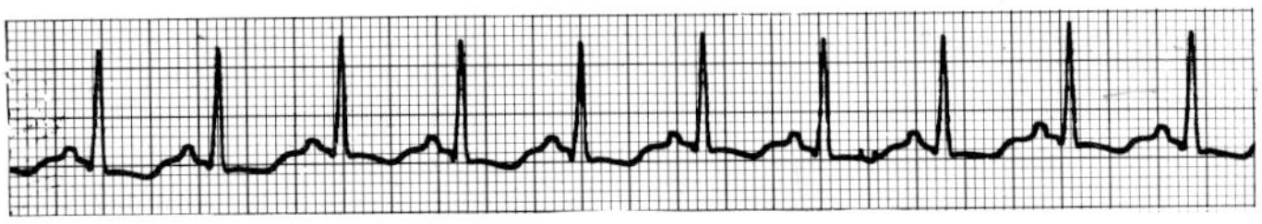

Let us review:

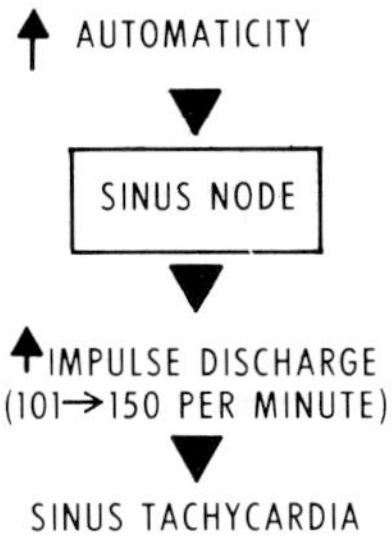

Fig. 5-6

89

29 Some factors have been identified as enhancing automaticity in the sinus node. In the setting of acute MI, the most significant factors are (1) sympathetic stimulation—fever, pain, anxiety; (2) heart failure; (3) hypoxia; (4) drugs—atropine, Isuprel, aminophylline. Initial therapy in the management of sinus tachycardia is directed toward correcting the *underlying cause* rather than depressing automaticity. For example, if the sinus tachycardia is associated with heart failure, initial therapy would be directed toward improving cardiac function and decreasing cardiac workload.

30 *Nursing orders:* The patient with sinus tachycardia
 1. Is patient symptomatic from the fast rate?
  — check blood pressure, sensorium, skin color, and temperature
 2. Is the tachycardia associated with heart failure?
  — auscultate lungs for rales
  — auscultate heart for gallop rhythms
  — check VCP readings and fluid balance
 3. Assess adequacy of oxygenation.
  — check skin color and temperature
  — observe character and rate of respirations
  — assess arterial blood gas values, especially pH, P_{CO_2}, and P_{O_2} levels
 4. Is the tachycardia associated with drug therapy?
  — Isuprel, atropine, aminophylline, epinephrine (Adrenalin), Dopamine
 5. Identify any stressors that may elicit a sympathetic response and thus increase the heart rate.
  — fever
  — pain
  — anxiety

Sinus bradycardia

31 When automaticity is depressed in the sinus node, the rate of impulse discharge from this area will *(increase/decrease)*. Slowing of the sinus rate below 60 beats per minute results in an arrhythmia known as sinus bradycardia.

decrease

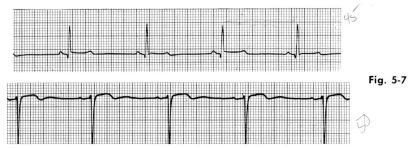

Fig. 5-7

32 *Let us review:*

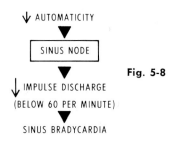

Fig. 5-8

33 Some factors have been identified as depressing automaticity and conduction in the sinus node. In the setting of acute MI, the most significant factors are: (1) ischemia (to the sinus node); (2) parasympathetic or vagal stimulation—ischemia to the vagal fibers, carotid sinus pressure, Valsalva maneuver; (3) drugs (digitalis, propranolol [Inderal]); (4) electrolyte imbalances (hyperkalemia). Sinus bradycardia is clinically significant *when* it causes a symptomatic fall in cardiac _____.

output

Remember: Cardiac output = _____ _____ × stroke volume

heart rate

Sinus bradycardias are also significant because *slow rates* may precipitate the development of dangerous tachyarrhythmias.
Initial therapy in the management of sinus bradycardia is directed toward *(accelerating/slowing)* the ventricular rate.

accelerating

34 *Nursing orders:* The patient with sinus bradycardia
  1. Is the patient symptomatic from the slow rates?
    — watch for the development of hypotension and sensorium changes
    — check for changes in skin color and temperature, diaphoresis
    — is patient having ventricular arrhythmias associated with the slow rate?
  2. Is the bradycardia associated with infarction of the inferior wall?
    Note: Slow rates classically accompany inferior wall myocardial infarction.
  3. Is the sinus bradycardia associated with any drug therapy?
    — is the patient receiving digitalis or propranolol?
  4. Is the patient hypoxic?
  5. Check serum K^+ levels
    Remember: Increased K^+ acts as a cardiac depressant.
  6. Have atropine at the bedside.
  7. Is bradycardia associated with Valsalva maneuvers or other vagal stimulation?

Sinus arrhythmia

35 The S-A node and the lungs are both innervated by the parasympathetic nervous system via the vagus nerve. The S-A node, therefore, *(may/may not)* be affected by respirations. The rate of the S-A node may *gradually* increase with inspiration and *gradually* decrease with expiration. If these effects are marked, the overall rhythm will appear *(regular/irregular)*. This irregularity is considered a *normal* physiologic process and is especially marked in young people.

may

irregular

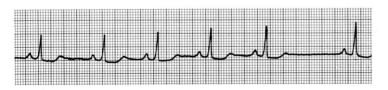

Fig. 5-9

Wandering pacemaker

36 The term *wandering pacemaker* is used to refer to a change in the pacemaker of the heart to another supraventricular focus. It usually occurs as a result of sinus slowing.

Remember: The lower portions of the atria and A-V junctional tissue have the property of automaticity. Therefore, they *(are/are not)* potential pacemakers of the heart.

are

If the lower portion of the atria gains control of the heart's rhythm, there will be a *change* in P wave morphology. This *may* be accompanied by a slight change in the P and QRS rates or P-R interval and is of minimal clinical significance.

Wandering Pacemaker

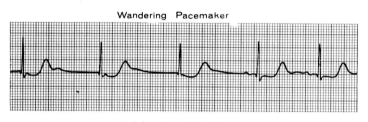

• Junctional to Sinus

Fig. 5-10

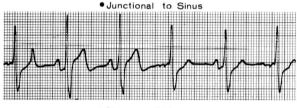

• Sinus to Atria

If the A-V junctional tissue gains control of the heart's rhythm, the P wave may disappear or become inverted on Lead II. There may be a significant decrease in ventricular rate. The clinical significance is identical to that of a junctional rhythm.

THE VENTRICULAR ARRHYTHMIAS

37 *Remember:* A ventricular arrhythmia is a manifestation of abnormal electrical activity in the _____.

ventricles

Some factors have been identified as contributing to the development of ventricular arrhythmias. In the setting of acute MI the most significant factors are: (1) electrical instability due to infarction, (2) hypokalemia, (3) hypoxia, (4) slow rates, (5) CHF, and (6) drugs (digitalis, Isuprel, aminophylline, Dopamine, epinephrine).

Ventricular arrhythmias produce a QRS complex that is *different* from the patient's normal complex and usually appears *(narrow/wide)*.

wide

Premature ventricular beats

38 An early sign of abnormal electrical activity in the ventricles is the appearance of *premature ventricular beats*. Premature beats are beats that occur before the next expected natural impulse has occurred. Premature ventricular beats occur before the next expected *(P/QRS complex)*.

QRS complex

The early, or premature, beats arise in the _____. Therefore, it can be expected that the QRS complexes of the premature beats will appear *different* from the patient's supraventricular beats and usually _____.

ventricles

wide

One early ventricular impulse is known as a *premature ventricular contraction* (PVC).

PVCs are also known as ventricular extrasystoles or ventricular ec- *anything after SA node* topic beats.

39 PVCs that arise from the same foci in the ventricles will have the same shape or morphology and are known as *unifocal PVCs*.

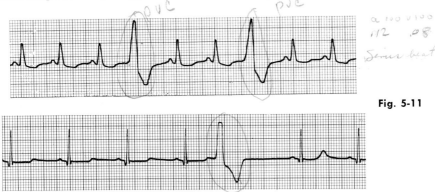

Fig. 5-11

PVCs that arise from different areas in the ventricles have different shapes and are known as *multifocal PVCs*.

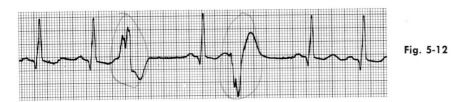

Fig. 5-12

40 PVCs may increase in frequency and appear every other beat. When a discharge sequence appears consisting of a sinus beat, a PVC, a sinus beat, a PVC, and so on, forming groups of two, the arrhythmia is known as *ventricular bigeminy*.

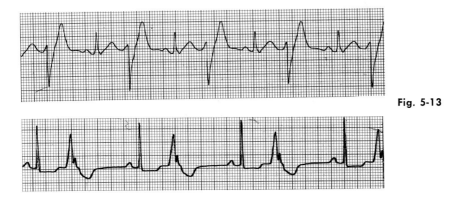

Fig. 5-13

Note: This is an arrhythmia commonly associated with digitalis toxicity.

41 The following are characteristics of PVCs, or *ventricular extrasystoles:* (1) they are *early,* or *premature;* (2) the QRS complexes of the premature beats are *different* from the patients' normal complexes and are usually wide; (3) they are *usually* but *not always* followed by a full compensatory pause.

When the pause following a premature beat is fully compensatory, the distance between the sinus beat that precedes the premature beat and the sinus beat that follows the premature beat is equal to the sum of two consecutive sinus intervals.

FULL COMPENSATORY PAUSE: PVC

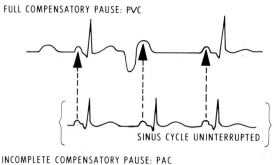

SINUS CYCLE UNINTERRUPTED

Fig. 5-14

INCOMPLETE COMPENSATORY PAUSE: PAC

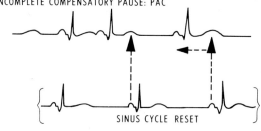

SINUS CYCLE RESET

42 PVCs are clinically significant because: (1) they are a manifestation of an underlying problem, and (2) they are often the precursors to more serious and life-threatening arrhythmias.

43 *Let us review:* PVCs are characteristically *(wide/narrow)* and/or   *wide*

_____ from the patient's normal beats. Other characteris-   *different*

tics of PVCs include: (1) they are *early* or _____ and   *premature*
(2) they are usually followed by a *full* compensatory pause.
PVCs that arise from different foci in the ventricles are known as

_____ PVCs.   *multifocal*
When a PVC occurs in a discharge sequence after every sinus beat,

the arrhythmia is known as ventricular _____.   *bigeminy*
PVCs are significant because they are often the *precursors* to the life-threatening arrhythmias.

Ventricular tachycardia

44 PVCs may increase in frequency until they begin to occur consecutively.
When three or more PVCs occur in a row, the arrhythmia is known as *ventricular tachycardia* (VT).
Note: Just *one* PVC can also initiate a run of VT.
Remember: The ventricles normally can initiate impulses at a rate

of 20 to _____ per minute.   *40*
A *ventricular* arrhythmia is known as a tachycardia when the ectopic ventricular rate is greater than *60* beats per minute.

45 Ventricular tachycardia has been classified into two types according to *rate.*
A ventricular tachycardia with a ventricular rate *greater than 60*

but *less than 100* beats per minute is known as *slow* ventricular tachycardia, as *nonparoxysmal* VT, or as an accelerated idioventricular rhythm.

A ventricular tachycardia with ventricular rate greater than 100 is known as *fast* or *paroxysmal* ventricular tachycardia.

This method of classification was developed because the *pathophysiology, clinical significance,* and *management* of these two types of ventricular tachycardia differ.

46 Let us first consider the pathophysiology and clinical significance of *slow* (or slower) *ventricular tachycardia.*

Slow ventricular tachycardia has a ventricular rate greater than

_____ but less than _____.   *60   100*

Slow ventricular tachycardia characteristically appears when the sinus rate slows.

Slow ventricular tachycardia is usually initiated by a "late" PVC or a ventricular escape beat. The term "late" PVC is used to describe those PVCs that occur late in diastole. They are also known as end-diastolic PVCs.

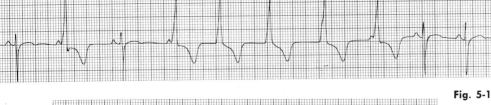

Fig. 5-15

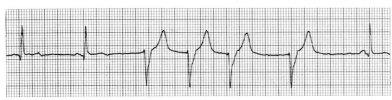

An escape beat is one that occurs because the next supraventricular impulse fails to appear.

Slow ventricular tachycardia results from increased automaticity

in the _____ and usually appears when the sinus rate   *ventricles*

_____.   *slows*

47 Slow ventricular tachycardia is generally a more *benign* arrhythmia than is fast VT. In some settings, however, it has the *potential for acceleration* and must be managed carefully. Frequently, it can be terminated by accelerating the *underlying bradyarrhythmias.*

In other settings the *ectopic focus* in the ventricles must be suppressed.

48 Let us now consider the pathophysiology and clinical significance of *fast* ventricular tachycardia.

Fast ventricular tachycardia, or paroxysmal VT, has an ectopic ven-

tricular rate greater than _____.   *100*

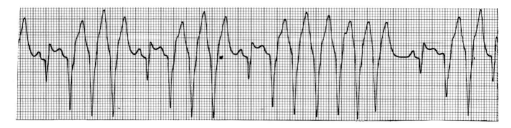

Fig. 5-16

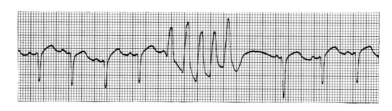

It may break through in spite of an adequate sinus rate and often comes suddenly. Fast VT is therefore also called *paroxysmal VT*.

Fast ventricular tachycardia is usually initiated by an "early" PVC. An "early" PVC is one that is so premature that it appears close to or on the T wave of the previous beat.

Remember: A stimulus that falls on the T wave may cause

_____ _____.   *repetitive firing*

49 Fast ventricular tachycardia is a malignant arrhythmia and frequently deteriorates into ventricular fibrillation.

Therapy is usually directed toward *depressing* the ectopic focus in the ventricles.

Note: If fast ventricular tachycardia appears in the setting of a slow rate, initial therapy may be directed toward accelerating the underlying bradyarrhythmia.

50 *Let us review:* Slow ventricular tachycardia has a rate greater than

_____ but less than _____ beats per minute. Fast ventricular tachy-   *60   100*

cardia has a rate greater than _____.   *100*

Slow ventricular tachycardia is usually initiated by a *(late/early)*   *late*

PVC.

Fast ventricular tachycardia, however, is *usually* initiated by a(n)

_____ PVC.   *early*

Slow ventricular tachycardia characteristically appears when the

sinus rate _____.   *slows*

Fast ventricular tachycardia, however, may appear in the presence of either fast or slow rates.

Slow ventricular tachycardia is clinically significant because it has

the potential for _____.   *acceleration*

Fast ventricular tachycardia is significant because it frequently de-

teriorates into _____ _____.   *ventricular fibril-*
                                                                              lation

Initial therapy in the management of *slow* ventricular tachycardia is usually directed toward accelerating the underlying

_____.   *bradyarrhythmia*

Initial therapy in the management of *fast* ventricular tachycardia is usually directed toward *depressing* the ectopic focus in the

_____.

Ventricular fibrillation

51 Ventricular fibrillation (VF) represents the most disintegrated

electrical activity that can occur in the _____.   *ventricles*
Ventricular fibrillation is usually initiated by a *single PVC* or a *run
of ventricular tachycardia.*
In the presence of ventricular fibrillation, the electrical activity is
so chaotic that the complexes have no distinct shape or morphology.

Thus in the presence of VF no distinct __QRS__ complexes will be   *QRS*
seen on the ECG.
The electrical activity is so disintegrated in this arrhythmia that
the heart cannot receive a signal to pump and *quivers ineffectually.*
As a result there is *no* cardiac output and clinical *death* occurs.

52 Ventricular fibrillation is divided into *two types* according to the
size of the fibrillatory waves.

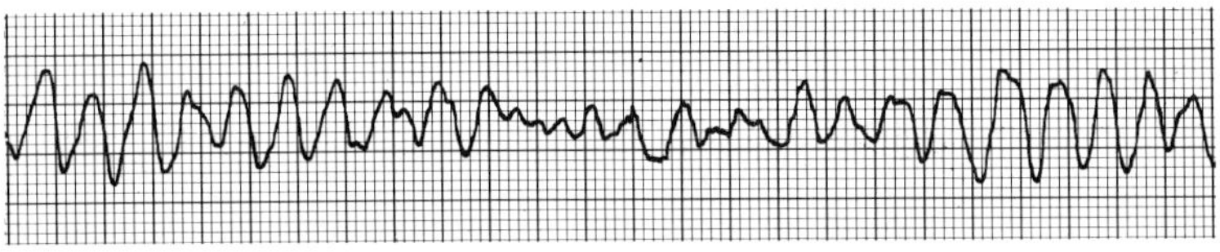

Fig. 5-17

In *coarse* VF the waves are of large amplitude.
Coarse VF implies that the fibrillation is of recent onset and that
electrical intervention will usually abolish the arrhythmia.
If coarse ventricular fibrillation is not terminated immediately, the
heart will become anoxic and depressed. The fibrillatory waves will
then become *fine.* Pharmacological and mechanical intervention is
then necessary before this arrhythmia will respond to electrical
therapy.

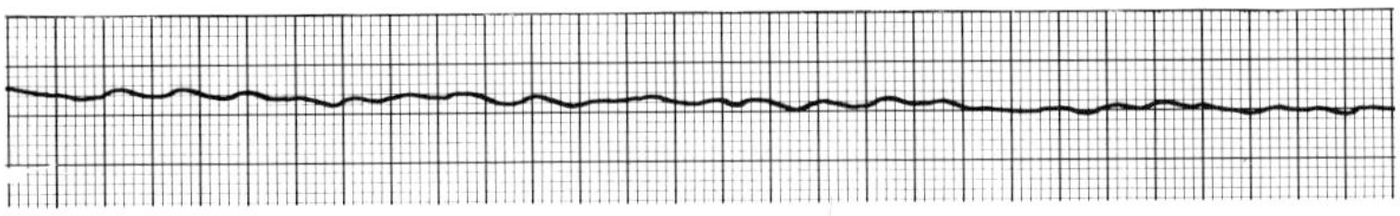

Fig. 5-18

53 *Let us review:* The most chaotic electrical activity that can occur

in the ventricles is known as _____ _____.   *ventricular fibrillation*

VF is usually intiated by a single __PVC__ or a run of   *PVC*

_____ _____.   *ventricular tachycardia*
In the presence of VF, distinct QRS complexes *(will/will not)* be   *will not*
seen on the ECG.
The electrical activity is so disintegrated in this arrhythmia that

the heart _____ ineffectually. As a result there is no   *quivers*

_____ _____ and _____ death occurs.   *cardiac output; clinical*

Coarse VF can usually be terminated by _____ intervention.   *electrical*

Fine VF, however, usually requires _____ and   *mechanical*

_____ intervention before it will respond to electri-   *pharmacological*
cal therapy.

54 *Nursing orders:* The patient with a ventricular arrhythmia
    1. Have lidocaine at the bedside.
    2. Medicate patient as necessary (according to institutional pol-
       icy).
    3. Evaluate the underlying causes.
       — in first 48 hours following infarction, ventricular arrhythmias
         are usually a result of electrical instability
       — check for hypokalemia
       — is patient hypoxic?
       — is arrhythmia arising in the presence of slow rates?
       — is patient receiving drugs such as Isuprel, Digoxin, amino-
         phylline, Dopamine?
       — is there evidence of heart failure?
    4. Make sure a cardioverter defibrillator is immediately available
       and in good working order.

Idioventricular rhythm

55 Let us now discuss another ventricular arrhythmia that usually ap-
    pears in the presence of depressed conduction.
    When conduction is depressed, the ventricles may assume control
    of the rhythm.
    Remember: Depressed conduction results in *(slow/fast)* rates. The   *slow*
    ventricles normally have the ability to initiate impulses at a rate of

    _____ to _____ per minute.   *20   40*

Fig.

    When the ventricles assume control of the rhythm at this rate, the
    arrhythmia is known as *idioventricular rhythm.*
    The QRS complex in the presence of *idioventricular* rhythm is usu-
    ally *(wide/narrow)* because it is originating in the ventricles.   *wide*

56 Idioventricular rhythm is clinically significant because: (1) it is
    slow and may cause a symptomatic fall in cardiac output, and (2)
    it may allow for the breakthrough of dangerous tachyarrhythmias.
    Initial therapy in the management of idioventricular rhythm is usu-
    ally directed toward *accelerating* the ventricular rate.

57 *Let us review:* When the ventricular rate of a ventricular
    rhythm is between 20 and 40, the arrhythmia is known as

    _____ _____.   *idioventricular*
    Idioventricular rhythm characteristically appears in the presence of   *rhythm*

    depressed _____.   *conduction*
    An idioventricular rhythm is clinically significant because: (1) it is

    slow and may result in a _____ fall in _____   *symptomatic; cardiac*

    _____, and (2) it may allow for the breakthrough of life-   *output*

    threatening _____.   *tachyarrhythmias*

98

THE ECTOPIC SUPRAVENTRICULAR ARRHYTHMIAS

58 Analysis of the QRS complex provides information about the origin

of the impulse: ventricular or _____. *supraventricular*
The term *supraventricular* implies that the origin of the impulse
is *(above/below)* the ventricles. *above*
Remember: Supraventricular impulses may arise in the _____ node, *S-A*
the _____, or the _____ _____ tissue. *atria; A-V junctional*
Supraventricular impulses *(are/are not)* usually transmitted *are*
through the normal conduction pathways to the ventricles. Therefore, supraventricular impulses will usually produce a *(narrow/* *narrow*
wide) QRS complex.
Thus the presence of a *narrow,* unchanging QRS complex can be
used as a guide when diagnosing a *(supraventricular/ventricular)* *supraventricular*
arrhythmia.
Analysis of the P *wave* and calculation of the *atrial rate* provides
the information for the differential diagnosis of supraventricular
arrhythmias.

Atrial arrhythmias

59 Atrial arrhythmias are a manifestation of abnormal electrical ac-

tivity in the _____. *atria*
Some factors have been identified as contributing to the development of atrial arrhythmias: In the setting of acute MI, the most
significant factors are: (1) atrial distention, as in heart failure;
(2) ischemia resulting from hypoxia or IWMI; (3) drugs (digitalis
toxicity); (4) pericarditis; (5) chronic disease of the sinus node.

60 *Remember:* When diagnosing supraventricular arrhythmias, the

_____ wave must be analyzed and the _____ rate calculated. *P   atrial*
When assessing supraventricular arrhythmias, it is necessary to lo-
cate the P waves. We suggest the following points be utilized when
locating P waves.
1. P waves are best visualized on Lead II.
2. P waves are small forces, and may be best seen when the amplitude, or gain, is increased.
3. Premature P waves are often hidden on the T wave of the previous beat. The T wave configuration of that beat should be
   compared to that of the patient's usual T waves.

Premature atrial beats

61 An early sign of abnormal electrical activity in the atria is the ap-
    pearance of *premature* atrial beats.
    Premature atrial impulses will appear on the ECG as *early P waves.*
    Remember: Atrial depolarization is represented on the ECG by the

_____ wave. *P*
A single early atrial impulse is known as a *premature atrial con-*
traction (PAC).
Note: PACs are also known as atrial extrasystoles and atrial ectopic beats. Throughout this discussion, these terms will be used in-
terchangeably.

62 Premature atrial contractions, or PACs, have these characteristic

features: (1) the P wave is early, or _____, and (2) the *premature*
P wave appears different from the normal sinus P wave on at least
one lead.

The P wave appears different from the normal sinus impulse because it is originating in the atria and not in the _____ node.

S-A

63 Premature atrial impulses are usually transmitted through the normal conduction pathways to the ventricles. Therefore, the premature P wave of a PAC *(is/is not)* usually followed by a QRS complex. The QRS complex produced is usually *(narrow/wide)* and/ or *(the same as/different from)* that of the basic rhythm.

is
narrow
the same as

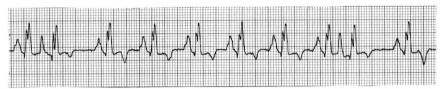

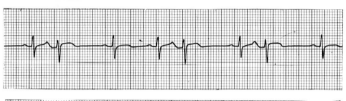

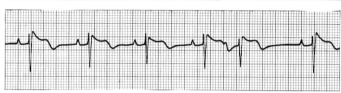

Fig. 5-20

64 If a premature atrial impulse finds the ventricles completely *refractory*, it *(will/will not)* be conducted through to the ventricles. Therefore, the P wave *(will/will not)* be conducted. The impulse is known as a nonconducted *PAC*. A nonconducted PAC will be seen

will not
will not

as a *(premature/late)* _____ wave that is not followed by a _____ complex.

premature; P; QRS

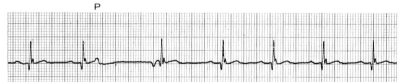

Fig. 5-21

65 If the premature atrial impulse finds the ventricles *partially* refractory, the impulse will be conducted with delay. A wider QRS complex conducted differently, or *aberrantly*, may follow the premature P wave. A PAC conducted in this manner is referred to as an aberrantly conducted PAC. (See Chapter 10.)

It is not unusual to see PACs conducted in any of these three ways in a given patient.

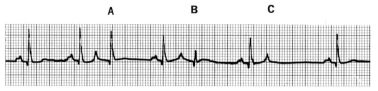

Fig. 5-22

A—conducted normally
B—conducted aberrantly
C—nonconducted
The criteria common to all of the above PACs is the premature ___ P wave.

Note: PACs may be conducted with normal, short, or long P-R intervals. Most commonly they are conducted with a P-R interval that is longer than normal because the ectopic atrial impulse finds the A-V node partially refractory.

Following a PAC, there is an *incomplete* compensatory pause because the ectopic atrial impulse prematurely discharges the sinus node and resets the sinus cycle. (See frame 41 for definition of a complete compensatory pause.)

66 Premature atrial contractions are clinically significant because: (1) they may indicate an underlying problem (in the setting of acute MI, they frequently indicate the presence of CHF), and (2) they may be precursors to more serious atrial arrhythmias.

Note: Just *one* PAC that falls during the vulnerable period of the atria may produce atrial flutter or fibrillation. PACs may increase in frequency and in this way also be *precursors* of atrial tachycardia, flutter, or fibrillation.

Atrial bigeminy

67 Premature atrial contractions may increase in frequency until they begin to occur consecutively. As they increase in frequency they may occur every other beat in a bigeminal pattern.

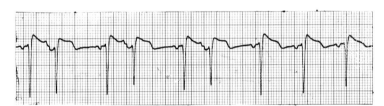

Fig. 5-23

Atrial tachycardia

68 When three or more PACs occur in a row, the arrhythmia is known as *atrial tachycardia.*

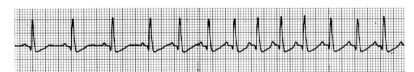

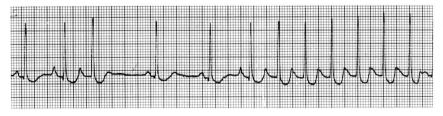

Fig. 5-24

Since this arrhythmia appears and disappears suddenly, it is frequently known as *paroxysmal atrial tachycardia (PAT).*
In atrial tachycardia, the atrial rate may range between 150 and

250 per minute. Characteristically, the atrial rate is in the lower range.

Remember: The atrial rate may be calculated by measuring the

_____ wave rate.   *P*

If the A-V node is functioning normally, every atrial impulse should

be conducted through to the _____.   *ventricles*

Therefore, in atrial tachycardia the ventricular rate will usually

be the same as the _____ rate.   *atrial*

69 If some of the atrial impulses are not conducted through to the ventricles, the arrhythmia is then known as *atrial tachycardia with block.*

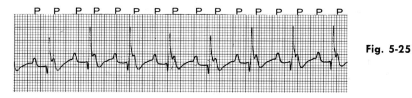

Fig. 5-25

Note: This arrhythmia is classically associated with digitalis toxicity.

Atrial flutter

70 An increase in the atrial rate lead to an arrhythmia known as *atrial flutter.* In atrial flutter, the atrial rate usually falls between 250 and 350 beats per minute.

In atrial flutter, the atria are initiating impulses so rapidly that this arrhythmia may assume a sawtooth appearance.

Note: This characteristic sawtooth pattern should not be relied upon when diagnosing atrial flutter; the atrial rate should first be measured.

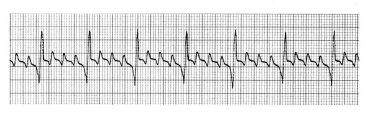

Fig. 5-26

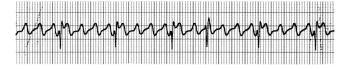

71 In atrial flutter, every atrial impulse is usually *not* conducted

through to the _____.   *ventricles*

The atria are discharging impulses so rapidly that even the healthy A-V node is not able to transmit all of the impulses.

Characteristically, the atrial rate in atrial flutter is approximately 300 per minute. Most commonly there is a 2 to 1 conduction ratio—every other impulse is conducted to the ventricles.

Thus there would be two P waves for every _____ complex. The   *QRS* ventricular rate would be half of the atrial rate, or approximately

_____. This arrhythmia is described as *atrial flutter with 2 to 1 conduction.*   150

Lead I

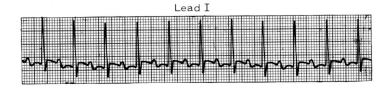

Lead AVF

Fig. 5-27

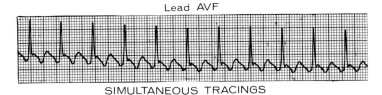

SIMULTANEOUS TRACINGS

Note: Detection of this arrhythmia is difficult because P waves may be hidden in the T waves. It is suggested that in the presence of a supraventricular arrhythmia with a ventricular rate of approximately 150 beats per minute the possibility of atrial flutter with 2 to 1 conduction should always be considered.

The conduction ratio may vary, depending on the adequacy of A-V conduction.

Note: It is important to record the rate of the ventricular response when diagnosing this arrhythmia.

Atrial fibrillation

72 The rate of impulse discharge from the atria may become faster and may result in an arrhythmia known as *atrial fibrillation.* In the presence of this rapid atrial rate, the shape or morphology of the

_____ waves will begin to deteriorate. At this point, the atria are   P
initiating imuplses so rapidly that a definite P wave rate can no longer be calculated.

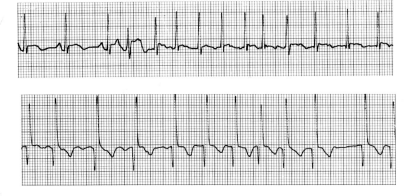

Fig. 5-28

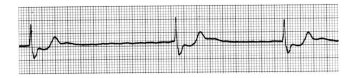

73 In the presence of atrial fibrillation, the A-V node is being bombarded with impulses. The A-V node selects and conducts impulses randomly. Therefore, in atrial fibrillation, the ventricular response will *always* be *(regular/irregular)*.

irregular

We suggest that, when a consistent P wave rate cannot be measured, in the presence of a supraventricular arrhythmia, and there is an irregular ventricular response, the arrhythmia be labelled *atrial fibrillation*.

Note: It is important to note the rate of the ventricular response when diagnosing this arrhythmia—for example, atrial fibrillation with a rapid ventricular response of 180.

74 IN SUMMARY: Atrial arrhythmias are clinically significant because:
1. They may result in a fast ventricular response, which will compromise cardiac output and thus decrease coronary blood flow, increase oxygen consumption of the myocardium, and may cause patient symptoms.
2. The atrial contribution to cardiac output may be lost.
3. They usually indicate an underlying problem.
   — CHF
   — pericarditis
   — ischemia
   — drug toxicity
   — sinus node dysfunction

Initial therapy in the management of persistent atrial tachycardia, atrial flutter, or atrial fibrillation is usually directed toward decreasing the ventricular rate. Subsequent therapy is directed toward correcting the underlying cause *and/or* depressing ectopic activity in the _____.

atria

75 *Nursing orders:* The patient with an atrial arrhythmia
1. Evaluate the *ventricular* response:
   — is the rate fast?
   — is the patient tolerating the fast rate?
   — check blood pressure, sensorium, skin color, and temperature
   — does the patient have coronary artery disease?
2. Assess patient for evidence of heart failure:
   — auscultate lungs for rales
   — auscultate heart for gallop rhythms
   — check VCP and fluid balance
3. Does the patient have evidence of pericarditis?
4. If rhythm is PAT with block, it is probably digitalis toxicity.
   — check serum potassium (K^+) level
5. Is drug therapy (Isuprel) associated with the arrhythmia?

Nodal or junctional arrhythmias

76 Nodal, or junctional, arrhythmias originate in the *A-V junctional* tissue. Junctional arrhythmias are therefore *(ventricular/supraventricular)*.

supraventricular

Remember: The differential diagnosis of suparventricular arrhythmias is dependent upon the analysis of the _____ wave. When a nodal, or junctional, arrhythmia occurs, the atria are depolarized in a reverse direction. This is known as *retrograde atrial* depolarization. Retrograde depolarization of the atria results in inversion of the

P

_____ wave. As a result, the P wave in Lead II appears *(negative/ positive)*.

P   negative

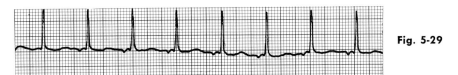

Fig. 5-29

In this type of arrhythmia, the P wave may be seen in *front* of or *behind* the QRS complex. The P wave may also become hidden

within the _____ complex.

QRS

77 Junctional arrhythmias can result from anything which (1) depress automaticity and conduction in the S-A node (for example, sinus bradycardia, digitalis); or (2) increases automaticity in the A-V junctional tissue (for example, digitalis intoxication, Isuprel).

78 Just as premature beats may originate in the atria, they may also originate in the A-V junctional tissue. Premature beats that originate in the A-V junctional tissue are known as premature junctional contractions (PJCs).

The following are characteristics of PJCs: (1) they are early, or premature, and (2) if a P wave is associated with the premature beat, it will be inverted or hidden.

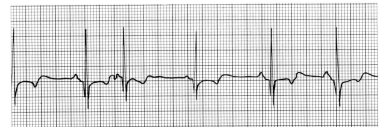

Fig. 5-30

Note: PJCs occur less frequently than PACs and are usually not clinically significant.

When the normal pacemaker in the S-A node is depressed, the A-V junctional tissue may assume control of the rhythm, and the rate is usually between 40 and 70 beats per minute. This is known as *idiojunctional* rhythm.

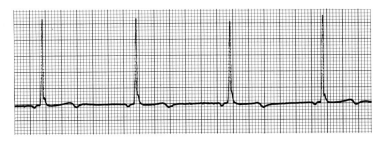

Fig. 5-31

When automaticity is enhanced in the A-V junctional tissue, the rhythm may again be controlled by the _____ node.

A-V

105

When this occurs, the ventricular rate is greater than 70 beats per minute and the arrhythmia is known as nodal, or junctional, tachycardia.

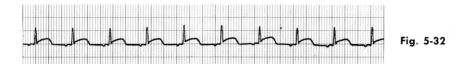

Fig. 5-32

79 Junctional arrhythmias are clinically significant when: (1) they indicate an underlying problem, (2) they are fast and compromise cardiac output and thus cardiac function, or (3) they are slow and result in a symptomatic fall in cardiac output.
Note: Cardiac output may be compromised because the atrial contribution may be lost.
Initial therapy in the management of junctional arrhythmias is usually directed toward: (1) correcting the underlying cause, (2) increasing the rate of the S-A node, and (3) depressing automaticity in the A-V junctional tissue.

80 *Nursing orders:* The patient with a junctional arrhythmia
1. Evaluate the ventricular response:
   — is the rate too fast or too slow?
   — check blood pressure, sensorium, skin color, and temperature
   — if patient is symptomatic because of a slow ventricular rate, have atropine at bedside
   — if patient is symptomatic because of junctional tachycardia with a fast ventricular response, have Dilantin available
2. Rule out digitalis toxicity.
Note: Digitalis intoxication is the most common cause of junctional tachycardia.

THE HEART BLOCKS

81 Let us now consider a group of arrhythmias that occur as a result of depressed conduction—the *heart blocks.*
Remember: The heart's conduction system allows for the rapid

transmission of electrical impulses from the _____ node, through ⟶ *S-A*

the ____ _____ tissue, to the _____. ⟶ *A-V junctional;*
An electrical impulse can be *delayed* or *blocked* at any point in this ⟶ *ventricles*
conduction system.
The group of arrhythmias that occur as a result of depressed con-

duction are known as heart _____. ⟶ *blocks*
Blocks may occur in any structure of the conduction system: the

_____ node, the _____ _____ tissue, or the bundle ⟶ *S-A; A-V junctional*

_____ system. ⟶ *branch*

Sinoatrial (S-A) block

82 Sinoatrial block occurs because conduction is depressed between

the sinus node and the _____. ⟶ *atria*
When sinoatrial block occurs, the normal sinus impulse is formed
but fails to reach the atria. As a result, the atria and the ventricles
(will/will not) be depolarized. ⟶ *will not*

Remember: Atrial depolarization is represented on the ECG by the

_____ wave. Ventricular depolarization is represented on the ECG   *P*

by the _____ complex.   *QRS*
Therefore, at the onset of a sinoatrial block, a _____ wave and a   *P*

_____ complex will suddenly be dropped.   *QRS*

83 When the *onset* of sinoatrial block is not recorded, it is difficult to
differentiate between this arrhythmia and *sinus bradycardia.*
When a sinus rate of 80 *suddenly* drops to 40, the arrhythmia is
most likely *sinoatrial block.* The pause in the rhythm associated
with an S-A block is usually equal to a multiple of original P
wave cycles.
Remember: Sinoatrial block is a manifestation of depressed *conduc-*

tion between the _____ node and the _____. *Sinus bradycardia* is   *S-A   atria*

a manifestation of depressed _____ in the sinus node.   *automaticity*
Another arrhythmia that may appear similarly on the ECG is *sinus
arrest,* which occurs when the sinus node is so depressed that no impulses are formed. Unlike an S-A block, the pause in the rhythm associated with a sinus arrest is of no predictable length.

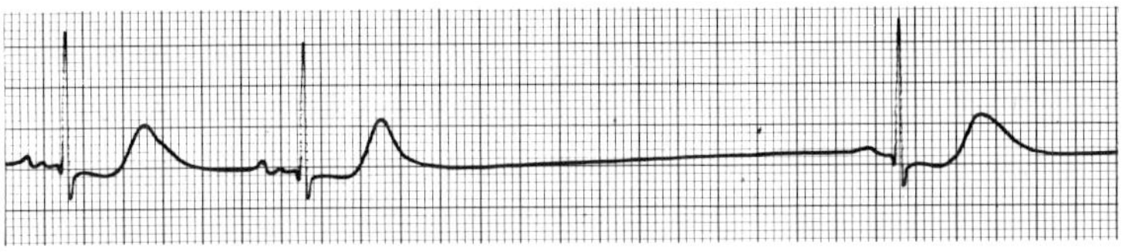

Fig. 5-33

84 Sinoatrial block and sinus arrest are potentially clinically significant because they may result in a *slow rate* and cause a symptomatic fall in cardiac output.
Therapy in the management of sinoatrial block is directed toward
accelerating conduction between the *sinus node* and the *atria.*
Therapy in the management of sinus arrest is directed toward en-

hancing _____ of the S-A node. Both therapeutic goals   *automaticity*
can usually be achieved with a single drug.

85 *Let us review:* Sinoatrial block is a manifestation of depressed con-

duction between the _____ node and the _____.   *S-A   atria*
When the sinus block occurs, the normal *sinus* impulse fails to

reach the _____.   *atria*
Sinus block is diagnosed on the ECG by the sudden absence of a

_____ wave and a _____.   *P   QRS*
If the onset of sinoatrial block is not recorded, it may be difficult

to distinguish between this arrhythmia and sinus _____   *bradycardia*
on the ECG.
Another arrhythmia that may appear as sinoatrial block on the

ECG is sinus _____.   *arrest*
Both sinus arrest and sinoatrial block are clinically significant when
they result in a sustained slow rate and thus cause a symptomatic

fall in _____ _____.   *cardiac output*

107

Therapy in the management of sinoatrial block is directed toward

accelerating conduction between the _____ node and the _____.   *S-A*   *atria*

A-V blocks

86 A-V blocks are a manifestation of depressed conduction between the
atria and the *ventricles*.
Therefore, in order to detect A-V blocks on the ECG, the _____   *P-R*
interval must be analyzed.
A-V blocks are classified according to (1) their location in relation
to the *His bundle,* and (2) their degree of pathology.
A-V blocks are classified as occurring either *above* or *below* the
His bundle.
A-V blocks that occur *above* the His bundle at the *A-V node* are
known as *supra-Hisian* blocks.
A-V blocks occurring *below* the His bundle in the *bundle branch
system* are known as *(supra-/infra-)*Hisian blocks.   *infra-*
A-V blocks are further classified into *three degrees* according to the
severity of the pathology.

First-degree A-V block

87 First-degree A-V block is a manifestation of *delayed conduction
time* between the sinus node and the ventricles. Although there is a
delay in conduction time, *all* impulses are conducted to the ventricles.
Remember: On the ECG the conduction time between the sinus

node and the ventricles is represented by the _____ interval.   *P-R*
In first-degree A-V block, the only abnormality on the ECG is a

prolonged _____ interval.   *P-R*
Remember: The normal P-R interval is from _____ to _____ second.   *0.12*   *0.20*
Therefore, a diagnosis of *first*-degree A-V block is made when the

P-R interval is greater than _____ second.   *0.20*
First-degree A-V block may occur as a result of pathology either
above or *below* the His bundle. To determine the location of the
block, the rhythm must be analyzed within the clinical setting in
which its occurs.

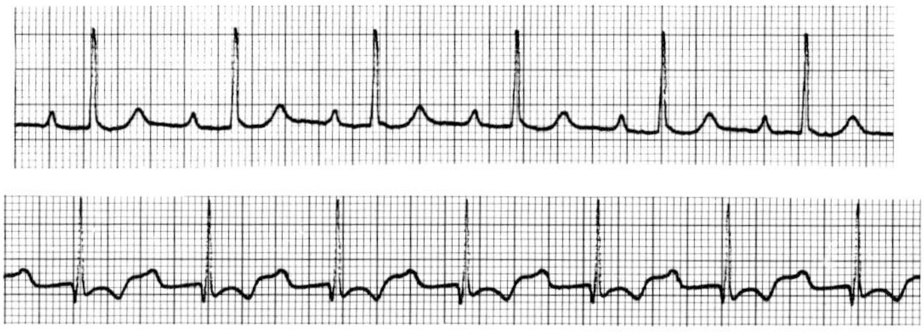

Fig. 5-34

88 *Let us review:* In first-degree A-V block, the sinus impulse is de-

layed in reaching the _____.   *ventricles*
First-degree A-V block is diagnosed on the ECG by the presence of
a *(prolonged/shortened)* P-R interval.   *prolonged*
In first-degree A-V block, each P wave *(will/will not)* be followed   *will*
by a QRS complex.

89 SUMMARY: *First-degree A-V block*

108

1. Sinus impulse delayed in reaching the ventricles.
2. May be a result of pathology *above* or *below* the His bundle.
3. P-R interval greater than 0.20 second.
4. Each P wave followed by a QRS complex.

Second-degree A-V block

90 When second-degree A-V block occurs, *one* or *more* sinus impulses
fail to activate the ventricles.
Atrial depolarization occurs normally, but ventricular depolarization *does not always* follow.
Therefore, in the presence of second-degree A-V block, P waves
(will/will not) be present. Each P wave, however, may not be fol-   *will*

lowed by a _____ complex.   *QRS*
ECG diagnosis of second-degree A-V block requires that there be
at *least* one *nonconducted* P wave or *"dropped"* QRS complex.
Remember: A-V blocks are classified according to their location in

relation to the _____ _____.   *His bundle*

91 Generally, *Type I*, or *Wenckebach*, second-degree A-V blocks occur
above the His bundle at the *A-V node*.
Note: These blocks are also known as *Mobitz I.*
Blocks of the *Wenckebach* type occur *(above/below)* the His bundle   *above*
at the A-V node.
Remember: The A-V node is primarily supplied by the *(right/left)*   *right*
coronary artery.
Blocks that occur at the *A-V node* are *usually* associated with *right*
coronary artery pathology.
Right coronary artery occlusion produces _____ wall MI.   *inferior*
Thus, second-degree A-V blocks of the Wenckebach type are associ-

ated with _____ wall MI.   *inferior*
Note: Wenckebach type second-degree A-V blocks may also occur as
a result of *digitalis toxicity* or chronic lesions of the conduction
system.
Wenckebach blocks occur in the presence of inferior wall MI as a

result of (1) ischemia to the _____ node, or (2) ischemia to the   *A-V*
parasympathetic (vagal) fibers that supply the A-V node.
In IWMI, the ischemia at the A-V node is *reversible.* Thus the A-V
blocks that occur as a result of this ischemia are *(transient/perma-*   *transient*
nent).
Second-degree A-V blocks of the Wenckebach type are thus described as being *ischemic* and *transient* in *nature.*

92 Type I (Wenckebach) block is diagnosed when a "dropped" QRS
is preceded by progressive *prolongation* of the P-R interval.
The progressive prolongation of the P-R interval eventually causes
the P wave to fall *in* the refractory period of the ventricles, and
thus a P wave eventually becomes blocked.

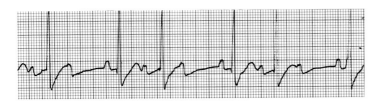

Fig. 5-35

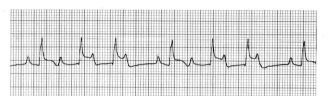

Fig. 5-35, cont'd

Note: In Fig. 5-35, strip No. 1, the block may be described as 3:2

Wenckebach because there are _____ P waves for every _____   *three*   *two*
QRS complexes.
Other characteristics of Type I, or Wenckebach, block are: (1)
constant P-P interval, and (2) irregular and decreasing R-R interval.

93   Wenckebach block is clinically significant because: (1) it may result in a slow rate and cause a symptomatic fall in cardiac output, and (2) it may be the precursor of third-degree A-V block.
Initial therapy in the management of second-degree A-V block of
the Wenckebach type is directed toward *accelerating (S-A/A-V)*   *A-V*
conduction.
Note: Because of its ischemic nature, Wenckebach block usually responds well to pharmacological intervention.

94   *Let us review:* Wenckebach is classified as a *(first-degree/second-*   *second-degree*
degree) A-V block and occurs *(above/below)* the His bundle at the   *above*

    _____ node.   *A-V*
Type I, or Wenckebach, blocks are associated with _____   *inferior*
wall MI.
Wenckebach blocks may also be a manifestation of _____ tox-   *digitalis*
icity.
Wenckebach classically occurs as a result of _____ to the   *ischemia*
A-V node and is *(transient/permanent)*.   *transient*
ECG diagnosis of Type I block requires the presence of: (1) pro-

gressive _____ interval prolongation preceding the "dropped" QRS,   *P-R*

(2) regular intervals between _____ waves, and (3) irregular inter-   *P*

vals between _____ waves.   *R*
Initial therapy in the management of Wenckebach is directed to-

ward accelerating _____ conduction.   *A-V*

95   Generally, Type II (Mobitz II) second-degree A-V blocks occur
below the His bundle in the *bundle branch system.*
Remember: The left coronary artery supplies most of the right bun-

dle branch and the anterosuperior division of the _____ branch.   *left*
The posteroinferior division of the left branch is also partially sup-

plied by the _____ coronary artery.   *left*
Blocks that occur *below the His bundle* are usually associated with
left coronary artery pathology.
Left coronary artery occlusion produces _____ wall MI.   *anterior*
Thus Type II, or Mobitz II, blocks may be associated with

_____ wall MI.   *anterior*
Note: Type II blocks may also occur as a result of *chronic lesions*
of the conduction system.

Type II (Mobitz II) blocks occur in anterior wall MI as a result of the *necrotic* process. In AWMI the blocks that occur in the bundle branch system may thus be described as being *necrotic* in *nature*.

96 Mobitz II block is diagnosed when a "dropped" QRS is seen which is *not* preceded by a progressive prolongation of the P-R interval. When this type of block occurs, the P-R interval remains fixed and the dropped beat occurs without warning.

Another characteristic of Type II second-degree A-V block is a regular interval between *P waves*.

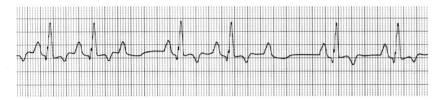

Fig. 5-36

97 Let us now consider the pathophysiology of Type II Mobitz block in more detail.

Remember: Type II block occurs as a result of pathology in the

_____ _____ system.   *bundle branch*

The bundle branch system is composed of *three fascicles:* the right

bundle branch, the anterosuperior division of the _____ branch,   *left*

and the _____ division of the _____ branch. (See   *posteroinferior   left*
Unit 6 for more details.)

A block in *one* of these fascicles is known as a *monofascicular* block.

A block in *two* of these fascicles is known as a *bifascicular* block.

A block in all *three* of these fascicles is known as a *trifascicular* block.

Type II second-degree A-V block usually occurs as a result of an *intermittent* trifascicular block.

98 When Type II block occurs, a sinus impulse fails to activate the ventricles because *all conduction pathways* between the His bundle

and the ventricles are _____.   *blocked*

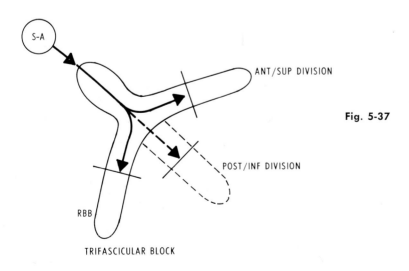

Fig. 5-37

TRIFASCICULAR BLOCK

Remember: ECG diagnosis of Mobitz II requires that there be a "dropped" *(P wave/QRS)* which is *not* preceded by progressive prolongation of the _____ interval.

QRS

P-R

In order to diagnose Type II, or Mobitz II, block, there must also *be evidence of preexisting bundle branch pathology.* It must be demonstrated that there is probability that trifascicular block is likely to occur.

There must be pathology in at least *two* of the three fascicles for it to be probable that the trifascicular or _____ block will occur.

Mobitz

Therefore, a bifascicular block in the presence of AWMI *(would/ would not)* be evidence that trifascicular block could occur.

would

The presence of a monofascicular block *(is/is not)* evidence that trifascicular block is *likely* to occur.

is not

99 Mobitz II is clincally significant because (1) it may be associated with a symptomatic fall in cardiac output, and (2) it is the precursor of third-degree, or complete, A-V block.

Initial therapy in the management of Type II second-degree A-V block is directed toward accelerating *(S-A/A-V)* conduction and thus the ventricular rate.

A-V

Note: Because the pathology in the bundle is necrotic in nature, Type II second-degree A-V block usually responds poorly to pharmacological intervention. Electrical intervention is usually necessary to manage this arrhythmia.

100 *Let us review:* Type II, or Mobitz II, block occurs as a result of pathology in the _____ _____ system.

bundle branch

Type II second-degree A-V blocks are associated with _____ wall MI.

anterior

Type II second-degree A-V block may also occur as a result of chronic lesions of the _____ _____.

conduction system

Type II second-degree A-V block usually occurs as a result of intermittent _____fascicular block.

tri-

In order to diagnose Type II, or Mobitz II, block on the ECG there must be:

1. a "fixed" P-R interval preceding the "dropped" _____ complex

QRS

2. regular intervals between _____ waves

P

3. evidence that the patient has preexisting _____ _____ pathology

bundle branch

Mobitz II is clinically significant when it is associated with a symptomatic fall in _____ _____.

cardiac output

Fixed ratio second-degree A-V block

101 Fixed ratio second-degree A-V block (for example, 2 to 1, 3 to 1, or 4 to 1) may be an end result of either a Wenckebach or a Mobitz II block. Unless the onset of the fixed ratio block is recorded, it is difficult to conclude if it is an end result of a Wenckebach or of a Mobitz II. Fixed ratio blocks should thus be analyzed in the clinical setting in which they occur.

In fixed ratio blocks that occur as an end result of a Wenckebach, the QRS complexes are generally *narrow.*

112

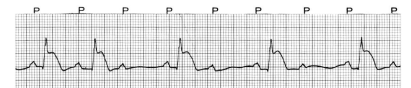

Fig. 5-38

In fixed ratio blocks that occur as an end result of a Mobitz, the QRS complexes are generally *wide*.

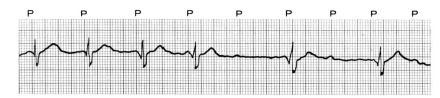

Fig. 5-39

102 IN SUMMARY:

Table 6. Second-degree A-V block (dropped QRS complex or nonconducted P waves)

Wenckebach (Type I)	Mobitz (Type II)
1. Lesion at A-V: supra-Hisian	1. Lesion in bundle branch system: infra-Hisian
2. Associated with: IWMI, digitalis toxicity, chronic lesion of conduction system	2. Associated with: AWMI, chronic lesions of the conduction system
3. Described as *ischemic, reversible,* and *transient*	3. Described as *necrotic* in nature
4. Dropped QRS preceded by progressive prolongation of the P-R	4. Dropped QRS preceded by a fixed P-R interval
5. Regular P-P intervals	5. Regular P-P intervals
6. Usually responds well to pharmacological intervention	6. Usually nonresponsive to pharmacological intervention and requires electrical intervention

103 *Let us review:* In *first-degree* A-V block all sinus impulses are

conducted to the ventricles but the conduction occurs with _____.   *delay*
In *second-degree* A-V block *some* of the sinus impulses fail to ac-

tivate the ventricles and some are _____.   *conducted*
The pathology involved in A-V block can progress in severity *until all sinus* impulses are blocked.
When this occurs, the A-V block is known as *third-degree,* or complete, *A-V block.*

Third-degree A-V block

104 In third-degree A-V block all of the sinus impulses fail to activate

the _____.   *ventricles*
There is no relationship between the *atria* and the *ventricles.*
Therefore, it can be expected that there will be no *fixed* relation-

ship between the _____ wave and the _____ complex.   *P*   *QRS*

Remember: The interval that denotes the relationship between the

atria and the ventricles is the _____ _____.   *P-R interval*
One of the characteristics of third-degree A-V block is a *highly
variable P-R interval.*

105 Third-degree A-V block may occur as an end result of Type I
(Wenckebach) second-degree A-V block.
Remember: Wenckebach occurs *(above/below)* the His bundle at   *above*

the _____ node.   *A-V*
When third-degree A-V block occurs following a Wenckebach, the
ventricles will usually be under the control of the A-V node and
the controlling rhythm will be *idiojunctional.*

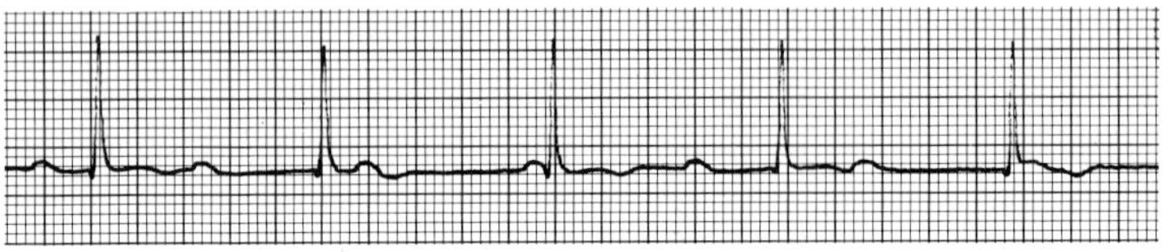

Fig. 5-40

Remember: The ventricular rate of an *idiojunctional* rhythm is

usually between 40 and _____ and the QRS complexes are *(narrow/*   *70*   *narrow*
wide) unless bundle branch block is present.

106 Third-degree A-V block may also occur as an end result of Type II
(Mobitz) second-degree A-V block.
Remember: Mobitz blocks occur *(above/below)* the His bundle in   *below*

the _____ _____ system.   *bundle branch*
When third-degree A-V block occurs following Type II block, the
ventricles will usually control the rhythm and the controlling
rhythm will be *idioventricular.*

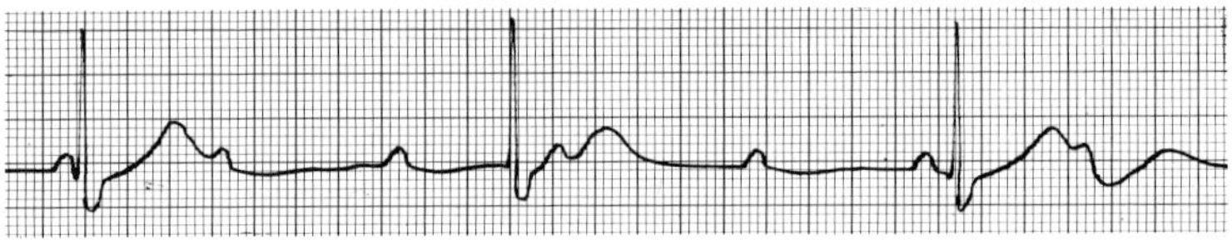

Fig. 5-41

Remember: The ventricular rate of an *idioventricular rhythm* is

usually between _____ and _____ and the QRS complexes are *(nar-*   *20*   *40*
row/wide).   *wide*

107 Third-degree, or complete, A-V block is clinically significant *when*
it is associated with a symptomatic fall in cardiac output.
Third-degree A-V block that occurs as an end result of a Mobitz
usually results in a symptomatic fall in cardiac output because

the ventricular rate is between _____ and _____.   *20*   *40*
Initial therapy in the management of third-degree A-V block is
directed toward accelerating A-V conduction and thus the

_____ rate.   *ventricular*

108 *Let us review:* When third-degree A-V block occurs, there is *no* re-

lationship between the _____ wave and the _____ complex.   *P*   *QRS*

As a result, there will be a highly variable _____ interval.   *P-R*

114

In the setting of acute MI, third-degree A-V block may occur
as an end result of Type I (_____) or Type II
(_____) second-degree A-V block.
When third-degree A-V block occurs as an end result of a Wenckebach, the rhythm controlling the ventricles will usually be

_____.
In idiojunctional rhythm, the VR is usually between ____ and ____
and the QRS complexes are usually *(wide/narrow)*.
When third-degree A-V block occurs as an end result of a
Mobitz, the rhythm controlling the ventricles will usually be

_____.
In idioventricular rhythm, the VR is *usually* between _____ and
_____ and the QRS complexes are usually *(wide/narrow)*.
Third-degree A-V block is clinically significant *when* it is associ-

ated with a symptomatic fall in _____ _____.

Wenckebach

Mobitz

idiojunctional
40   70
narrow

idioventricular
20
40   wide

cardiac output

109 SUMMARY: *Third-degree A-V block*
1. No relationship between P waves and QRS complexes.
2. Highly variable P-R interval.
3. Regular P-P intervals.
4. Regular R-R intervals.
5. Following Wenckebach block, controlling rhythm will usually
   be *idiojunctional*.
6. Following Mobitz block, controlling rhythm will usually be *idioventricular*.

110 *Nursing orders:* The patient with an A-V block
1. Is the *A-V block* resulting in symptomatic bradycardia?
2. Identify the type of MI the A-V block is associated with.
3. If A-V block is associated with inferior wall MI:
   — have atropine at the bedside
     Remember: A-V blocks associated with inferior wall MI are
     ischemic in nature and usually respond well to pharmacologi-
     cal intervention.
   — watch for the development of Type I (Wenckebach) second-
     degree A-V block
   — watch for the development of third-degree A-V block with
     idiojunctional rhythm
4. If A-V block is associated with anterior wall MI:
   — first-degree A-V block
     — monitor the patient for the development of intraventricu-
       lar conduction disturbances (see Unit 6)
     — observe for the development of Mobitz II block
   — in anticipation of Type II (Mobitz) block
     — have Isuprel drip on standby
     — have pacemaker on standby
   — watch for the development of third-degree A-V block with
     idioventricular rhythm

THE CLINICAL SIGNIFICANCE OF ARRHYTHMIAS

111 Arrhythmias become potentially life-threatening under three conditions: (1) when they originate in the *ventricles*, (2) when they
result in a critically *slow* rate, and (3) when they result in a critically *fast* rate.

Therefore, the three most significant types of arrhythmias are:

(1) the _____ arrhythmias, (2) the _____arrhyth-   *ventricular   brady-*
mias, and (3) the fast supraventricular arrhythmias.

112 Ventricular arrhythmias are clinically significant because they

may result in ventricular tachycardia or ventricular _____.   *fibrillation*
Ventricular tachycardia is clinically significant because it may re-

sult in a symptomatic fall in _____ _____, or it may lead   *cardiac output*

to _____ _____.   *ventricular fibrillation*
Ventricular fibrillation is clinically significant because it is essen-

tially a state of no _____ _____, or clinical _____.   *cardiac output;*
                                                                       death

113 Bradyarrhythmias are clinically significant when: (1) they result
in a symptomatic fall in cardiac output, or (2) they allow for the
breakthrough of dangerous tachyarrhythmias.
Bradyarrhythmias may cause a fall in cardiac output because:

Cardiac output = stroke volume × _____.   *heart rate*
The following symptoms reflect a significant fall in cardiac output:
1. hypotension (cold, clammy skin)
2. sensorium changes
3. left ventricular failure
4. a fall in urinary output

114 Fast supraventricular arrhythmias are clinically significant when
they result in a *fall* in cardiac output and compromise cardiac
function.
Tachyarrhythmias may decrease cardiac output by shortening ventricular filling time in *(systole/diastole)*.   *diastole*
The coronary arteries receive their blood supply during *diastole*.
In the presence of tachyarrhythmias, therefore, coronary blood
flow may be reduced.
Fast supraventricular arrhythmias may decrease cardiac output
by: (1) *(decreasing/increasing)* ventricular filling time, and (2)   *decreasing*
(decreasing/increasing) coronary blood flow.   *decreasing*

115 Initial therapy in the management of ventricular arrhythmias is

directed toward depressing _____ _____ in the ventri-   *ectopic activity*
cles. Subsequent therapy would be directed toward correcting the

_____ cause.   *underlying*
In the setting of acute MI, ventricular arrhythmias are most com-

monly a manifestation of: (1) electrical _____ due to   *instability*

ischemic areas, (2) electrolyte imbalance (hypo-_____),   *kalemia*

and (3) drug _____.   *toxicity*
Initial therapy in the management of bradyarrhythmias is di-

rected toward accelerating the _____ _____.   *ventricular rate*
Remember: The most common cause of bradyarrhythmias in the
setting of a coronary care unit is probably *inferior wall MI*.
Initial therapy in the management of fast supraventricular ar-

rhythmias is directed toward decreasing the _____   *ventricular*

_____.   *rate*

116

Subsequent therapy may be directed toward depressing _____ *atrial*

automaticity and correcting the _____ cause. *underlying*
Remember: The most common cause of fast supraventricular ar-

rhythmias in the setting of acute MI is _____ _____. *heart failure*

116 *Nursing orders:* Arrhythmias
1. Anticipate and be prepared for *bradyarrhythmias* and *ventricular* arrhythmias in the first 48 hours.
   — In anticipation of bradyarrhythmia, have atropine, Isuprel, and equipment for pacemaker insertion available.
   — In anticipation of ventricular arrhythmias, have lidocaine, Pronestyl, Dilantin, Inderal, and equipment for countershock available.
2. If life-threatening arrhythmias should occur, immediate *intravenous* therapy will be required. Therefore, make certain the patient has a patent IV at all times.
3. Monitor for the effects of drugs, electrolyte imbalances, hypoxic states, and any changes in the QRS morphology.
   — Verify any changes in the QRS morphology with a standard twelve-lead ECG.
4. When an arrhythmia occurs, observe how the patient is *tolerating* the arrhythmia. Report:
   — changes in sensorium
   — changes in skin color and temperature
   — change in the rate or character of respirations
   — hypotension
   — left ventricular failure—rales, gallops
   — decrease in urinary output
5. Record on ECG strip an example of any arrhythmia; if possible record the *initiating factor.*
6. Investigate the *underlying cause* of any arrhythmia. For example, in the presence of a rapid supraventricular arrhythmia in acute MI, check for signs of CHF.
7. In anticipation of life-threatening arrhythmias, have resuscitation equipment and emergency drugs *immediately* available.

Equipment	*Drugs*
Ambu or Hope bag and mask with oxygen catheter	Sodium bicarbonate
Airways	Calcium chloride
Wall and portable oxygen and suction	Adrenalin (1:10,000)
Endotracheal tubes	Xylocaine
Laryngoscope	Atropine
Arrest board	Isuprel
Countershock machine	Pronestyl
Blood gas syringes	Levophed
	Aramine
	IV solutions of 5% dextrose in water

Suggested readings

Andreoli, K. G., and others: Comprehensive cardiac care, ed. 3, St. Louis, 1975, The C. V. Mosby Co.

Asevedo, I. M., Watanabe, Y., and Driefus, L. S.: Reassessment of A-V junctional rhythms, Heart Lung 1(5):626, Sept.-Oct. 1972.

Bashour, F. A., Jones, E., and Edmonson, R.: Cardiac arrhythmias in acute MI. II. Incidence of the common arrhythmias with special reference to ventricular tachycardia, Dis. Chest 51: 520, 1967.

Castellanos, A., Ghafour, A. G., and Soffer, A.:

Digitalis-induced arrhythmias; recognition and therapy, Cardiov. Ther. 1:108, 1969.

Castellanos, A., Lemberg, L., and Arcebal, A. G.: Mechanisms of slow ventricular tachycardias, Dis. Chest 56:470, 1969.

Castellanos, A., and others: Post-infarction conduction disturbances; a self-teaching program, Dis. Chest 56:421, 1969.

Castellanos, A., Spence, M., and Chapell, D.: Management of ventricular standstill, Rocom Monitor, June, 1970.

Chon, L. J., Donoso, E., and Friedberg, C. K.: Ventricular tachycardia, Prog. Cardiov. Dis. 9: 29, 1966.

Damato, A. N., and Lau, S. H.: Clinical value of the electrogram of the conduction system, Prog. Cardiov. Dis. 13:119, 1970.

DePasquale, N. P.: The electrocardiogram in complicated acute myocardial infarction, Prog. Cardiov. Dis. 13:1, 1970.

Dubin, D.: Rapid interpretation of EKG's, Tampa, Fla., 1970, Cover Publishing Co.

Fisch, C.: Electrophysiologic basis of clinical arrhythmias, Heart Lung 3(1):51, Jan.-Feb. 1974.

Fisch, C.: Self assessment—aberrant conduction, Heart Lung 2(2):260, Mar.-Apr. 1973.

Friedberg, C. K., Cohen, H., and Donoso, E.: Advanced heart block as a complication of acute MI; role of pacemaker therapy, Prog. Cardiov. Dis. 10:466, 1968.

Gozensky, C., and Thorne, D.: Rabbit ears: An aid in distinguishing ventricular ectopy from aberration, Heart Lung 3(4):634, July-Aug. 1974.

Grace, W. J., and Keyloun, V.: The coronary care unit, New York, 1970, Appleton-Century-Crofts.

Guyton, A. C.: Textbook of medical physiology, Philadelphia, 1971, W. B. Saunders Co.

Hecht, H. H.: Atrioventricular and intraventricular conduction: Revised nomenclature and concepts, Am. J. Cardiol. 31:232, Feb. 1973.

Hoffman, B. F., Cranefield, P. F., and Wallace, A. G.: Physiological basis of cardiac arrhythmias, Mod. Concepts Cardiov. Dis. 35:107, 1966.

Hurst, W. J., and Logue, R. B., editors: The heart arteries and veins, New York, 1970, McGraw-Hill Book Co.

Hurst, W. J., and Myerberg, R. J.: Cardiac arrhythmias; evolving concepts, I, Mod. Concepts Cardiov. Dis. 37:73, 1968.

Hurst, W. J., and Myerberg, R. J.: Cardiac arrhythmias; evolving concepts, II. Mod. Concepts Cardiov. Dis. 37:79, 1968.

Kimball, J. T., and Killip, T.: Aggressive treatment of arrhythmia in acute MI; procedures and results, Prog. Cardiov. Dis. 10:483, 1968.

Langendorf, R., and Pick, A.: Atrioventricular block, its nature and clinical significance, Circulation 38:819-821, 1968.

Lemberg, L., Castellanos, A., and Arcebal, A.: The treatment of arrhythmias following acute myocardial infarction, Med. Clin. N. Am. 55: 273, 1971.

Marriott, H. J. L.: Differential diagnosis of supraventricular and ventricular tachycardia, Geriatrics Nov. 1970.

Marriott, H. J. L.: Practical electrocardiography, Baltimore, 1968, The Williams & Wilkins Co.

Mazzolini, A.: Electrophysiologic mechanisms of sudden death in patients with coronary artery disease, Heart Lung 2(6):841, Nov.-Dec. 1973.

Moe, G. K., and Mendez, C.: Physiologic basis of premature beats and sustained tachyarrhythmias, New Eng. J. Med. Feb. 1, 1973.

Netter, F. H.: Heart—The Ciba Collection of Medical Illustrations, Summit, N. J., 1969, Ciba Publications.

Noble, R. J.: An approach to supraventricular tachycardias, Heart Lung 3(1):64, Jan.-Feb. 1974.

Pick, A.: Mechanisms of cardiac arrhythmias from hypothesis to physiologic fact, Am. Heart J., Aug. 1973.

Rosen, K., and others: Site of heart block in acute myocardial infarction, Circulation 42:925, 1970.

Schamroth, L.: Idioventricular tachycardia, Dis. Chest 56:466, 1969.

Schamroth, L.: An introduction to electrocardiography, Edinburgh, 1971, Blackwell Scientific Publications.

Schamroth, L.: The disorders of cardiac rhythm, Edinburgh, 1971, Blackwell Scientific Publications.

Scherf, D.: Remarks on the nomenclature of cardiac arrhythmias, Prog. Cardiov. Dis. 13:1, 1970.

Segal, I., and Schamroth, L.: The basic forms of reciprocal rhythm, Heart Lung 2(5):732, Sept.-Oct. 1973.

Singer, D. H., and Geneick, R. E.: Electrophysiologic aspects of aberrancy, Am. J. Cardiol. Vol. 28, Oct. 1971.

Singer, D. H., and Teneick, R. E.: Pharmacology of cardiac arrhythmias. In Friedberg, C. K., editor: Current status of drugs in cardiovascular disease, New York, 1969, Grune & Stratton, Inc.

Surawicz, B.: Ventricular fibrillation, Am. J. Cardiol. Vol. 28, Sept. 1971.

Vassalli, M.: Automaticity and automatic rhythms, Am. J. Cardiol. Vol. 26, Sept. 1971.

Wit, A. L., Rosen, M. R., and Hoffman, B. F.: Electrophysiology and pharmacology of cardiac arrhythmias. Relationship of normal and abnormal electrical activity of cardiac fibers to the genesis of arrhythmias. B. Re-entry Section 1, Am. Heart J. 88(5):664, Nov. 1974.

The intraventricular conduction disturbances

1 The intraventricular conduction system has three main components: the *His bundle,* the *right bundle branch,* and the *main left
branch.* The main left branch subdivides into two fascicles: the *anterosuperior* and the *posteroinferior.*
The components of the intraventricular conduction system are best
visualized in the *horizontal plane.*

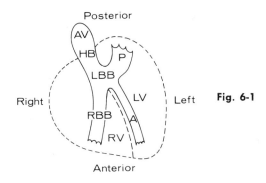

Fig. 6-1

2 *Remember:* The borders of the horizontal plane are _____,   *anterior*

_____, _____, and _____.   *posterior; right; left*
Note: In this plane, the anterosuperior division of the left bundle

lies _____. The posteroinferior division of the left bun-   *anteriorly*

dle lies _____.   *posteriorly*

DEFINITIONS

3 Let us now define some terms commonly used when discussing
blocks in the intraventricular conduction system.
The term *bundle branch* will be used when referring to the major
branches of the intraventricular conduction system.
The major branches of the intraventricular conduction system are:

the _____ _____ _____ and the _____ _____   *right bundle branch;*
                                                                main left branch
_____.

Blocks that occur in the major branches are known as _____   *bundle*

_____ blocks.   *branch*
Examples of bundle branch blocks are: right bundle branch block
(RBBB) and left bundle branch block (LBBB).

4 Blocks that occur in half of the left branch are known as *hemiblocks.*
The term hemiblocks, therefore, refers to a block in either the

_____ or _____ division of the left bun-   *anterosuperior;*
dle.   *posteroinferior*

A block in the anterosuperior division is known as *left anterior hemiblock (LAH)*.

A block in the posteroinferior division is known as *left posterior hemiblock (LPH)*.

5 In this discussion, the term *fascicle* will be used when referring to any branch of the intraventricular conduction system.

The *fascicles* of the intraventricular conduction system are: the

_____ _____ _____ and the _____   *right bundle branch;*
                                                                          anterosuperior

and _____ divisions of the main left branch.   *posteroinferior*

6 Blocks that occur in the fascicles are known as _____   *fascicular*
blocks.

Fascicular blocks can further be described according to the number of fascicles involved.

7 A block in *one* fascicle is called a monofascicular block. Examples of monofascicular blocks are: LAH, LPH, and RBBB.

A block in *two* fascicles is called a *bifascicular* block. Examples of bifascicular blocks are: RBBB and LAH; RBBB and LPH.

A block of *three* fascicles is called a _____fascicular block. An ex-   *tri-*
ample of trifascicular block is RBBB, LAH, and LPH occurring together.

NORMAL VENTRICULAR ACTIVATION

8 Before discussing blocks that occur in the intraventricular conduction system, let us first review *normal ventricular activation*.

The first part of the ventricles to be depolarized is the _____.   *septum*

The septum is normally activated from *left* to *right* and _____   *posteriorly*

to _____.   *anteriorly*
Depolarization of the septum produces the small *(q/r)* wave seen in   *r*
Lead V_1 and the small *(q/r)* seen in Lead V_6.   *q*
The waves of depolarization then spread through both the *right* and
left ventricles.

9 *Remember:* The left ventricle lies posteriorly. Therefore, the sum
of all electrical forces traveling through the ventricles is a force

shifted slightly to the _____ and _____.   *left*   *posteriorly*

THE MAIN LEFT BRANCH (LBB) AND COMPLETE LEFT
BUNDLE BRANCH BLOCK (CLBBB)

10 Each branch of the intraventricular conduction system and its associated conduction disturbance will now be considered. The main left
branch emerges from the bundle of His and lies against the septum.
Septal depolarization is normally initiated in this area. Two fascicles are emitted from the main left branch. The main left bundle
may be compared with the trunk of a tree. The anterosuperior and
posteroinferior fascicles are analogous to the branches of this tree.
The main left bundle is supplied by both the *right* and *left* coronary
arteries. Although the main left bundle can be blocked as a result
of acute myocardial infarction, a more common cause of complete
left bundle branch block is *sclerosis*, or calcification, of this area.

11
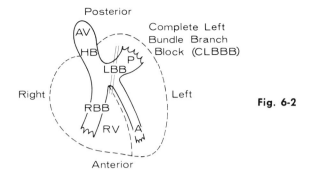

Posterior

Complete Left
Bundle Branch
Block (CLBBB)

Fig. 6-2

12 In the presence of complete left bundle branch block (CLBBB), there is *abnormal* septal depolarization.
Remember: Normal septal depolarization occurs from _____ to   *left*

_____. In CLBBB, the septum is depolarized from _____ to   *right*   *right*

_____. This results in a loss of the *small r wave* in Lead _____   *left* V_1

and of the *small q wave* in Lead _____. V_6

13 In the presence of CLBBB, the only fascicle still conducting impulses to the ventricles is the _____ bundle branch. Therefore,   *right*
the ventricles are activated through this branch.

14 When ventricular activation occurs in this way, the impulse is *delayed* in reaching the left ventricle. It can then be expected that, in the presence of CLBBB, the QRS will be *(narrow/wide)*. This delay   *wide*
is seen on the ECG as a *medial* change in the QRS complex. *Medial*
means the delay is seen in the *(middle/last)* portion of the QRS   *middle*
complex.

15 Bundle branch blocks are best visualized in the *horizontal* plane.
Leads V_1 and V_6 are used in the ECG diagnosis of bundle branch blocks.

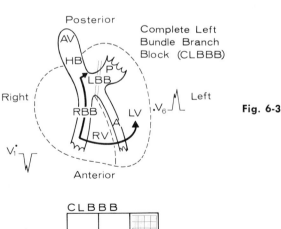

Posterior

Complete Left
Bundle Branch
Block (CLBBB)

Fig. 6-3

16
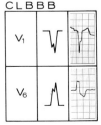

CLBBB

Fig. 6-4

THE RIGHT BUNDLE BRANCH (RBB) AND RIGHT
BUNDLE BRANCH BLOCK (RBBB)

17 The right bundle branch and the anterosuperior division of the left bundle exist in a common portion of the septum for a short segment. Then the right bundle emerges as a thin, singular fascicle.

18 The right bundle branch is primarily supplied by the left coronary artery.
Remember: The left coronary artery supplies the *(inferior/anterior)* surface of the left ventricle. It can then be anticipated that right bundle branch (RBBB) will be seen most frequently in the presence of *(anterior/inferior)* wall myocardial infarction.

anterior

anterior

19

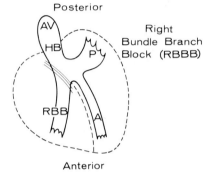

Fig. 6-5

20 When right bundle branch block (RBBB) occurs, septal depolarization is usually not altered. Septal depolarization occurs normally

from _____ to _____. Therefore, the small r wave in Lead V$_1$ and the small q in Lead V$_6$ *(will/will not)* be seen.

left   *right*

will

21 In the presence of RBBB the only fascicle still conducting impulses

to the ventricles is the _____ bundle branch. Therefore, ventricular activation occurs *through* the *left bundle branch*. In RBBB, the left ventricle is activated normally, but the *right ventricle is* activated with *delay*.
This delay is seen on the ECG as a *terminal* change in the QRS. Terminal delays occurs in the *(middle/last)* portion of the QRS complex.

left

last

22 *Remember:* Bundle branch blocks are best visualized in the horizontal plane. Therefore, Leads V$_1$ and V$_6$ are also used to diagnose RBBB on the ECG.

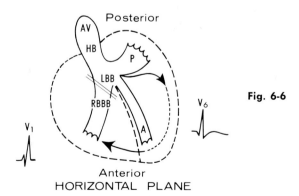

Fig. 6-6

HORIZONTAL PLANE

23 *Note:* If the septal forces are lost, as in anteroseptal myocardial infarction, the small r in Lead V_1 and small q in Lead V_6 will not be present. The QRS will then assume a qR configuration in Lead V_1 rather than the classic rSR′ pattern shown in the example below. However, it will still be a predominantly upright complex in Lead V_1 exhibiting terminal delay.

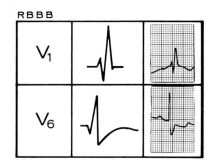

Fig. 6-7

24 SUMMARY: *The right bundle branch*
 1. Singular blood supply—left coronary artery
 2. RBBB commonly occurs in the presence of *anterior* wall myocardial infarction
 3. Characteristics of RBBB: septal depolarization usually not altered; terminal delay—slurring and widening of S wave in Lead V_6; rSR′ or qR configuration in Lead V_1 (predominantly upright complex).

THE HEMIBLOCKS

25 The main left branch subdivides into two fascicles: the

_____ division and the _____ division.   *anterosuperior;*
It is possible that a conduction block may occur in only *half* of   *posteroinferior*
the left bundle. The term used to describe these "half blocks" is

_____.   *hemiblock*

26 When a hemiblock occurs, there are still normal conduction pathways to the ventricles. Therefore, in the presence of hemiblocks only minimal changes in the QRS duration are seen on the ECG. However, hemiblocks do cause shifts in the *electrical axis of the heart.* Therefore, before considering the identification of hemiblocks on the ECG, we will discuss a method for calculating the *electrical axis.*

Calculating the electrical axis

27 *Let us review:* Axis is defined as the summation force, or summa-

tion _____.   *vector*
Remember: The left ventricle has *(more/less)* electrical forces than   *more*
does the right ventricle. Therefore, in the normal adult the axis is
shifted toward the *(right/left).*   *left*

28 The electrical axis is usually considered and calculated in the *frontal plane.*
Remember: The limb leads are derived in the _____ plane.   *frontal*

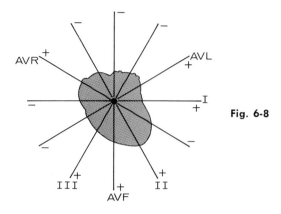

Fig. 6-8

29 This reference system can be divided into four quadrants, with Leads I and aVF serving as coordinates.

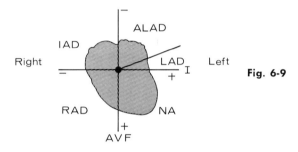

Fig. 6-9

30 If the electrical axis lies within the lower left quadrant, the axis

is _____ (NA).   *normal*

If the axis deviates toward the lower *right* quadrant, it is consid-

ered to be _____ axis deviation (RAD).   *right*

If the axis deviates toward the upper *left* quadrant, it is considered

to be _____ axis deviation (LAD).   *left*

Left axis deviation is further subdivided into *left axis* and *abnormal left axis*. *Abnormal left axis deviation* (ALAD) occurs when the axis is shifted far to the left.

If the heart's electrical forces deviate toward the *upper right* quadrant, the axis is considered to be *indeterminate* axis deviation (IAD).

31 The coordinates may be joined by a circle, and degrees assigned as reference points.

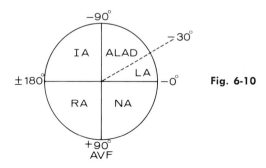

Fig. 6-10

124

32 Normal axis lies between ±0° and +_____. $90°$

Right axis lies between +90° and +_____. $180°$

Left axis lies between ±0° and −_____. $90°$

Abnormal left axis lies between −30° and −_____. $90°$

Indeterminate axis lies between +_____ and +_____. $180°$ $240°$

33 For the purposes of this discussion, it is not necessary to learn the degrees presented in each quadrant. It is more important to assess the QRS *morphology* in the presence of normal and abnormal axis and determine why the axis shifts in different clinical settings.

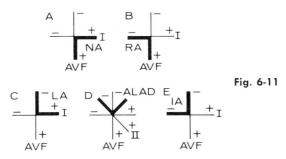

Fig. 6-11

34 When the axis is within *normal* limits, the net ventricular forces travel toward both the *(positive/negative)* pole of Lead I and toward the *(positive/negative)* pole of Lead aVF. *positive*
positive
The QRS complex, therefore, should be *(positive/negative)* in Lead I and *(positive/negative)* in Lead aVF when the axis is normal. *positive*
positive

35 When the axis is shifted to the right, the QRS complex is *(positive/negative)* in Lead I and *(positive/negative)* in Lead aVF. *negative*   *positive*

36 When the axis is shifted to the left, the QRS complex is *(positive/negative)* in Lead I and *(positive/negative)* in Lead aVF. *positive*
negative

37 When diagnosing *abnormal left axis,* we must consider the QRS morphology in Lead II as well as in Leads I and aVF. When the axis is *abnormal left,* the QRS complex is *(positive/negative)* in Lead I and *(positive/negative)* in Leads II and aVF. *positive*
negative

38 When the axis is indeterminate, the QRS complex is *(positive/negative)* in Lead I and *(positive/negative)* in Lead aVF. *negative*
negative

39 The clinical causes of axis deviation in the setting of acute myocardial infarction will be presented in the remainder of this chapter. We have given special emphasis to axis deviation and hemiblocks.

40 IN SUMMARY:

	I	AVF	II
NA			
RA			
LA			
ALAD			
IA			

Fig. 6-12

125

Left anterior hemiblock (LAH)

41 The anterosuperior division of the left bundle branch has a common anatomical origin with the _____ bundle branch.   *right*
Thus these two fascicles are often injured simultaneously.

42 The anterosuperior division is supplied by the *(left/right)* coronary artery. Thus the anterosuperior division will commonly be involved in infarctions of the *(anterior/inferior)* wall.   *left*

    anterior

43 The anterosuperior division of the left bundle is thought to be the *most* vulnerable structure of the intraventricular conduction system. This vulnerability is due to: (1) anatomical location in the hemodynamically turbulent aortic area, (2) its thinness and length,

and (3) its singular blood supply—the _____ coronary artery.   *left*

44 A block of the anterosuperior division of the left bundle is known as

_____ _____ _____ _____.   *left anterior hemi-*
    block (LAH)

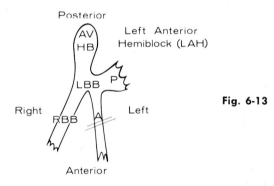

Fig. 6-13

45 ECG diagnosis of *hemiblocks* is made on the basis of *axis* shifts.
In the presence of LAH, the axis shifts to abnormal left.
Remember: when abnormal left axis deviation occurs, the QRS complex is *(positive/negative)* in Lead I and *(positive/negative)* in Leads II and aVF.   *positive*   *negative*

46 Let us now consider *the reasons why* the axis shifts to abnormal left in the presence of LAH. We will also derive the specific QRS patterns associated with this conduction disturbance.

47 The electrical axis is calculated by examining Leads I, _____, and   *II*

_____. *Remember:* these leads are derived in the *frontal*   *aVF*
plane.
Therefore, to understand the axis shifts associated with hemiblocks, we must visualize the intraventricular conduction system in the frontal plane.

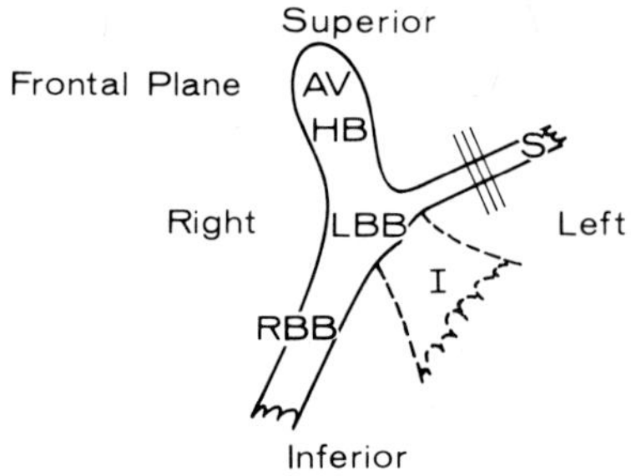

Fig. 6-14

48 As seen in the frontal plane, the anterosuperior division of the left bundle lies *(inferiorly/superiorly)*. The *posteroinferior* division lies *(inferiorly/superiorly)*.

When the *anterosuperior* division of the left bundle is blocked (LAH), activation of the left ventricle occurs through the *posteroinferior* division of the left bundle.

49 Because activation occurs through the *posteroinferior* division, the initial forces in LAH are shifted *inferiorly* and to the right. This *initial* force produces small r waves in Leads II and aVF and a small q in Lead I.

Remember: Leads II and aVF reflect the electrical activity of the *inferior* wall.

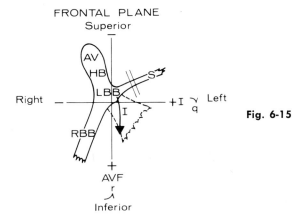

Fig. 6-15

50 The *main* forces then shift *superiorly* and to the *left*. These forces produce deep S waves in Leads II and aVF and a large R wave in Lead I.

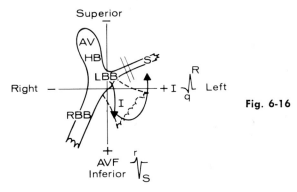

Fig. 6-16

51 Because the *main* forces are shifted superiorly and to the left, in LAH the axis shifts to *abnormal* left.

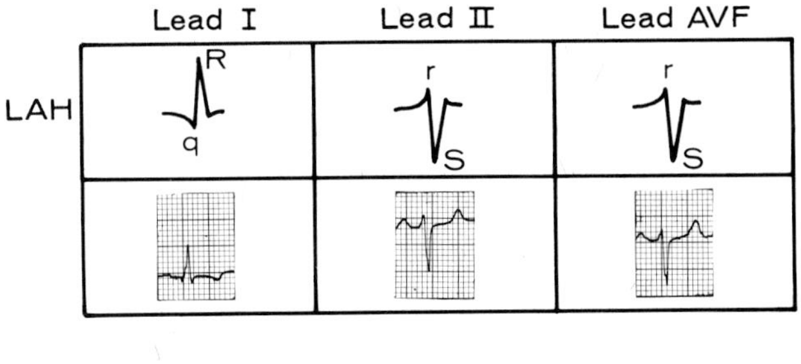

	Lead I	Lead II	Lead AVF
LAH			

Fig. 6-17

127

52 Another cause of abnormal left axis deviation (ALAD) is *inferior* wall myocardial infarction.

It is important to differentiate between the QRS patterns seen in inferior wall myocardial infarction and LAH.

In both IWMI and LAH, Lead I is *(positive/negative)* and Leads II and aVF are *(positive/negative)*. However, the morphology of the QRS complexes in these two settings differs.

positive
negative

53 In inferior wall myocardial infarction, Leads II and aVF are negative and assume a *large Q, small r* configuration (Qr). Lead I is positive and has a *small q, large R* configuration (qR).

Note: The large Q waves in Leads II and aVF represent necrosis of tissue in the *(anterior/inferior)* wall.

inferior

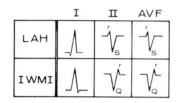

Fig. 6-18

Note: In LAH, Leads II and aVF are *(positive/negative)* and the QRS has a(n) _____ configuration. In IWMI, Leads II and aVF are again *(positive/negative)*, but the QRS has a(n) _____ configuration. In both settings Lead I is *(positive/negative)*.

negative
rS
negative   *Qr*
positive

54 Other causes of *ALAD* include right apical pacing, left ventricular pacing via the middle cardiac vein, Wolff-Parkinson-White syndrome Type B, hyperkalemia, severe chronic obstructive pulmonary disease, and left coronary arteriography.

55 *Let us review:* LAH most commonly occurs in combination with *(RBBB/LAH)*. LAH plus RBBB are known as a _____ block. LAH and RBBB are most frequently seen in the presence of _____ wall myocardial infarction.

In order to diagnose LAH on the ECG, there must be *(LAD/ALAD)*. When LAH occurs, the QRS is *(positive/negative)* in Lead I and *(positive/negative)* in Leads II and aVF. There are also specific QRS patterns in LAH. In Leads II and aVF, the QRS assumes a(n) *(rS/Qr)* configuration.

RBBB; bifascicular

anterior

ALAD   *positive*
negative

rS

56 SUMMARY: *Left anterior hemiblock (LAH)*
1. Anterior division supplied by left coronary artery—LAH seen in setting of *anterior* wall myocardial infarction.
2. LAH often accompanies RBBB.
3. ECG diagnosis of LAH:
   — there must be ALAD.
   — Lead *I* is positive; Leads II and aVF are negative
   — Lead *I*—qR configuration
   — Lead *II*—aVF-rS configuration

Left posterior hemiblock (LPH)

57 The posteroinferior division of the left bundle branch is the first fascicle emitted from the His bundle. It appears as the true continuation of the main left branch because of its thickness.

58 The posteroinferior division of the left bundle is supplied by both

the _____ and _____ coronary arteries.   *right   left*

59 The posteroinferior division of the left bundle is the *least* vulnerable structure of the intraventricular system. This fact is attributed
to its: (1) anatomical location in a hemodynamically nonturbulent
area, (2) thickness and length, and (3) dual blood supply—the

_____ and _____ coronary arteries.   *right   left*

60 A block of the posterior division of the left bundle is known as

_____ _____ _____ _____.   *left posterior hemi-*
                                                                       block (LPH)

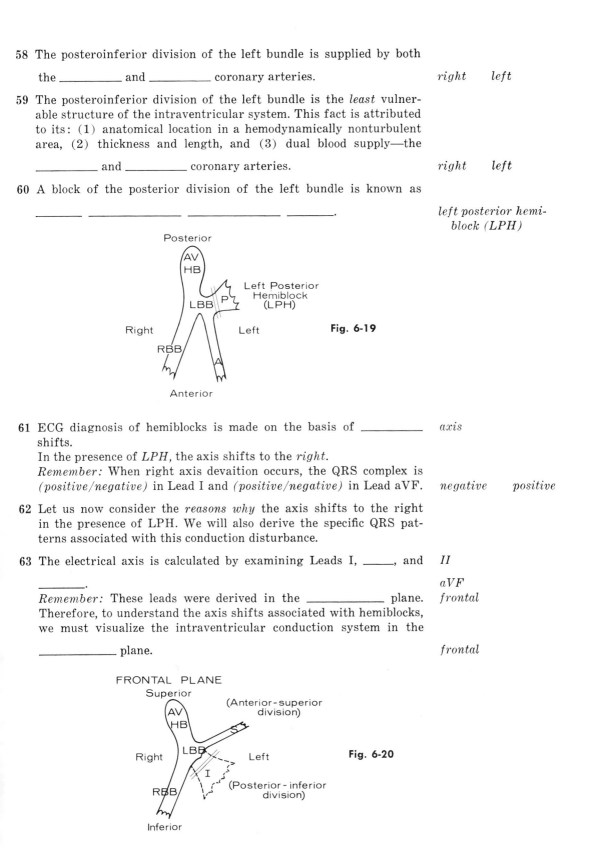

Fig. 6-19

61 ECG diagnosis of hemiblocks is made on the basis of _____   *axis*
shifts.
In the presence of *LPH*, the axis shifts to the *right*.
Remember: When right axis deviation occurs, the QRS complex is
(positive/negative) in Lead I and *(positive/negative)* in Lead aVF.   *negative   positive*

62 Let us now consider the *reasons why* the axis shifts to the right
in the presence of LPH. We will also derive the specific QRS patterns associated with this conduction disturbance.

63 The electrical axis is calculated by examining Leads I, _____, and   *II*

_____.   *aVF*
Remember: These leads were derived in the _____ plane.   *frontal*
Therefore, to understand the axis shifts associated with hemiblocks,
we must visualize the intraventricular conduction system in the

_____ plane.   *frontal*

FRONTAL PLANE

Fig. 6-20

64 In the frontal plane, the *posteroinferior* division of the left bundle

129

lies *(inferiorly/superiorly)*. The anterosuperior division lies

_____.

When the *posteroinferior* division of the left bundle is blocked (LPH), activation of the left ventricle occurs through the

_____ division of the left bundle.

inferiorly

superiorly

anterosuperior

65 Because activation occurs through the *anterosuperior* division, the *initial* forces in LPH are shifted *superiorly* and to the left.
This *initial* force produces a *small q* wave in Lead aVF and a *small r* wave in Lead I.

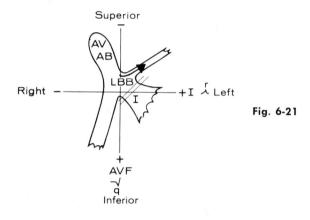

Fig. 6-21

66 The *main* forces, then, shift *inferiorly* and to the *right*. These forces produce large R waves in Leads II and aVF.
Remember: Leads II and aVF reflect the electrical activity of the

_____ wall of the left ventricle.

inferior

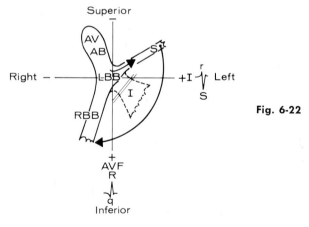

Fig. 6-22

67 Because the *main* forces are shifted *inferiorly* and to the *right*, in the presence of LPH the axis shifts to the *right*.
Note: LPH is the *exact* mirror image of LAH.

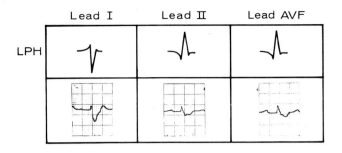

	Lead I	Lead II	Lead AVF
LPH			

Fig. 6-23

68 Another cause of right axis deviation (RAD) is *lateral* wall MI. It is important to differentiate between the QRS patterns seen in lateral wall myocardial infarction and LPH.
In both LWMI and LPH, Lead I is *(positive/negative)* and Leads II and aVF are *(positive/negative)*. However, the morphologies of the QRS complexes in these two settings *differ*.

negative
positive

69 In lateral wall myocardial infarction, Lead I is negative and assumes a *large Q, small r* configuration (Qr). Leads II and aVF are positive and have a small q, large R configuration (qR).
Note: The large Q wave in Lead I represents necrosis of tissue in the *(lateral/inferior)* wall.

lateral

	I	AVF	II
LPH			
LWMI			

Fig. 6-24

Note: In LPH, Lead I is negative and the QRS has a(n) ＿＿＿ configuration. In LWMI, Lead I is also negative, but the QRS has a(n)

rS

＿＿＿ configuration. In both settings Leads II and aVF are *(positive/negative)*.

Qr   *positive*

70 LPH cannot be diagnosed on the ECG unless other causes of RAD are excluded: right ventricular hypertrophy, chronic lung disease, pulmonary emboli, Wolff-Parkinson-White syndrome Type A, right ventricular pacing via the outflow tract, left ventricular pacing via the great cardiac vein, dextrocardia, right coronary arteriography.

71 *Let us review:* LPH is often seen in combination with *(RBBB/ LAH)*. When LPH occurs, it indicates *(mild/severe)* coronary artery disease. The ECG diagnosis of LPH is dependent upon the presence of *(RAD/ALAD)*. In the presence of LPH, the QRS is *(positive/negative)* in Lead I and *(positive/negative)* in Leads II and aVF.
The QRS in Lead I assumes a(n) *(rS/Qr)* configuration. In Leads II and aVF the QRS assumes a(n) *(rS/qR)* configuration.

RBBB
severe

RAD
negative   *positive*

rS
qR

72 SUMMARY: *Left posterior hemiblock*
  1. Posterior division is supplied by both the ＿＿＿ and ＿＿＿ coronary arteries. LPH indicates severe coronary artery disease.

right   *left*

  2. LPH is usually seen in combination with ＿＿＿＿.

RBBB

3. ECG diagnosis of LPH:
— there must be RAD
— Lead I is negative; Leads II and aVF are positive
— Lead I—rS configuration;
— Leads II and aVF—qR configuration.

73

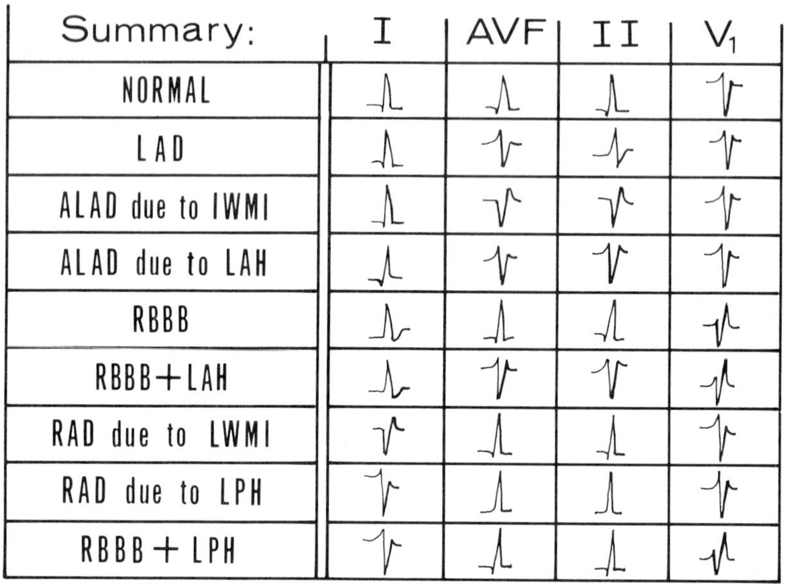

Summary:	I	AVF	II	V₁
NORMAL				
LAD				
ALAD due to IWMI				
ALAD due to LAH				
RBBB				
RBBB+LAH				
RAD due to LWMI				
RAD due to LPH				
RBBB + LPH				

Fig. 6-25

Implications for nurses

74 Bundle branch blocks and hemiblocks are clinically significant because they are the precursors of symptomatic Type II, or Mobitz II,
A-V blocks (see Unit 5).
Remember: Type II blocks usually occur as a result of *(right/left)*   *left*
coronary artery pathology and are associated with infarctions of

the _____ wall.   *anterior*

75 *Let us review:* A block that occurs in *one* fascicle is known as a

_____fascicular block. Examples of monofascicular blocks are   *mono-*

_____, _____, and _____.   *RBBB   LAH   LPH*
A block that occurs in *two* fascicles is known as a _____fascicular   *bi-*

block. Examples of bifascicular blocks are _____ plus _____   *RBBB   LAH*

and _____ plus _____.   *RBBB   LPH*
A block that occurs in *three* fascicles is known as a _____fascicular   *tri-*
block. A trifascicular block occurs when the RBBB and the

_____ and _____ divisions of the left bundle are   *anterior; posterior*
blocked simultaneously.

76 Trifascicular block may occur transiently or may be permanent.
Type II (Mobitz) second degree A-V block occurs as a result of a

transient, or intermittent, _____fascicular block.   *tri-*
Complete heart block may be a manifestation of *sustained* trifascicular block.

132

77 Symptomatic A-V block is usually preceded by the development of bundle branch blocks and hemiblocks.
Nurses who can diagnose bundle branch blocks and hemiblocks can anticipate the development of symptomatic A-V block.

78 Evidence of pathology in *two* of the three fascicles demonstrates that there is probability that trifascicular block may occur. *Note:* In bifascicular block, there is only one *fascicle* still conducting im-

pulses to the _____.   *ventricles*
Therefore, a bifascicular block in the presence of AWMI *(is/is not)*   *is*
evidence that trifascicular block could occur.

79 In the setting of AWMI, bifascicular block is usually a result of *RBBB and LAH. Remember:* AWMI is associated with *(right/left)*   *left*
coronary pathology. Both the RBB and the anterior division of the

left bundle are supplied by the _____ coronary artery.   *left*
Note: LPH may also occur in the presence of extensive AWMI and diffuse coronary artery disease.

80 Therefore, in the presence of AWMI, the nurse should monitor the

patient for the development of _____ and _____ because   *RBBB   LAH*
these blocks frequently occur together. Bifascicular blocks *(may/*   *may*
may not) be precursors of symptomatic A-V block.
RBBB is diagnosed by a change in the QRS morphology in Leads

_____ or _____. V_1 V_6
LAH is diagnosed by the development of _____ and changes in   *ALAD*
the QRS morphology.

81 If no fascicular blocks are present in the setting of AWMI, the patient should be monitored on either Lead II or V_1. If LAH occurs,

the development of an ALAD can best be observed on Lead _____. If   *II*

RBBB develops it can best be observed on Lead _____. V_1

82 In the presence of RBBB, the patient should be observed for the de-

velopment of _____. Therefore, this patient should be monitored   *LAH*

on Lead _____.   *II*

83 In the presence of either LPH or LAH, the patient should be ob-

served for the development of _____. Therefore, the patient   *RBBB*

should be monitored on Lead _____. V_1

84 In the presence of a bifascicular block, the patient should be monitored closely for any further conduction abnormalities. *Remember:*

In bifascicular block there is(are) only _____ fascicle(s) still con-   *one*
ducting impulses to the ventricles.
When a bifascicular block occurs suddenly, the nurse should notify the physician, prepare an Isuprel drip, and prepare for prophylactic pacemaker insertion.

85 *Let us review:* Bifascicular blocks may be precursors of the devel-

opment of _____fascicular block. In the setting of AWMI, the most   *tri-*

common type of bifascicular block is _____ plus _____.   *RBBB   LAH*

Transient trifascicular block became apparent as Type II or

_____ A-V block. Sustained trifascicular block may also ap-   *Mobitz*

pear as _____ _____ A-V block.   *third-degree (complete)*
The development of symptomatic A-V block may be observed for by

monitoring the patient for _____fascicular blocks.   *bi-*

86 *Nursing orders:*
   1. Place chest electrodes in the same position or as near the same
      position as possible each day. If electrodes are changed, note on
      hourly rhythm strips.
   2. If gain (size of complex) is changed for any reason, note on
      hourly rhythm strips.
   3. If no fascicular blocks are present, monitor the patient on Lead
      II or V_1.
   4. In the presence of RBBB, monitor the patient on Lead II to ob-
      serve for the development of LAH.
   5. In the presence of LPH or LAH, monitor the patient on Lead V_1
      to observe for the development of RBBB.
   6. In the presence of bifascicular block (such as RBBB plus LAH
      or RBBB plus LPH) monitor the patient closely for conduction
      abnormalities (such as first-degree A-V block, second-degree
      A-V block [Mobitz II], or complete A-V block). Monitor on what-
      ever lead shows both clear p waves and QRS complexes so that
      A-V block may be more easily detected.
   7. When a bifascicular block occurs suddenly, and in the setting of
      AWMI, the nurse should: (a) notify the physician immediately,
      (b) prepare an Isuprel drip on stand-by, and (c) prepare for
      pacemaker insertion.
   8. If no fascicular blocks are present in the setting of AWMI, the
      patient should be monitored on Lead II or V_1. If LAH occurs,
      the development of an ALAD can best be observed on Lead _____.   *II*
      If RBBB develops, it can best be observed on Lead _____.   *V_1*
   9. In addition to continuous monitoring, documentation of Leads I,
      II, aVF, and V_1 should be made every 4 hours. This will allow the
      nurse to make a more comprehensive analysis of the intraventric-
      ular conduction system.

ECTOPY ASSOCIATED WITH BUNDLE BRANCH BLOCK
AND FASCICULAR BLOCK PATTERNS

87 The QRS patterns associated with bundle branch blocks and hemiblocks are important not only in predicting the onset of A-V blocks,
   but also in determining the origin of ventricular ectopy.
   The V leads are used to diagnose conditions in which there are dif-
   ferences in the time between right and left ventricular activation.
   Remember: The V leads were used in the diagnosis of bundle branch
   blocks.
   The V leads may also be used to determine the origin of ventricular
   ectopy.

Right ventricular ectopy

88 *Let us review:* When an impulse is blocked in the LBB, the QRS in
   Lead V_1 is *(positive/negative)* and *(narrow/wide)*.   *negative   wide*
   Depolarization of the left ventricle occurs across the ventricular
   (conduction tissue/muscle tissue) and this accounts for the width   *muscle tissue*
   of the QRS complex.

89 When a ventricular ectopic beat originates in the *right ventricular*
    His-Purkinje tissue, the impulse activates the left ventricular mus-
    cle without first activating the LBB. The LBB is not physiologi-
    cally blocked, but activation occurs in such a way that this pathway
    is not used. Thus the resulting QRS pattern associated with right

    ventricular ectopy is similar to that which occurs in _____ bundle   *left*
    branch block.

    The predominant forces travel from right to left *(away from/*   *away from*
    toward) Lead V$_1$ and across the ventricular muscle tissue resulting
    in a *(positive/negative)* and *(wide/narrow)* complex in this lead.   *negative*   *wide*

RV ECTOPY

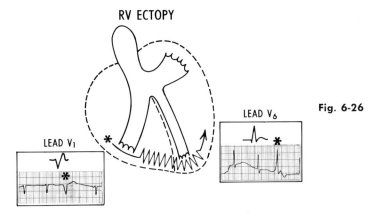

Fig. 6-26

Left ventricular ectopy

90 *Let us review:* When an impulse is blocked in the RBB, the QRS in
    Lead V$_1$ is *(positive/negative)* and *(narrow/wide)*.   *positive*   *wide*
    Depolarization of the right ventricle occurs across the ventricular
    (conduction tissue/muscle tissue), and this accounts for the width   *muscle tissue*
    of the QRS complex.

91 When a ventricular ectopic beat originates in the *left ventricular*
    His-Purkinje tissue, the impulse activates the right ventricular
    muscle without first activating the RBB. The RBB is not physio-
    logically blocked, but activation occurs in such a way that this path-
    way is not used. The resulting QRS pattern associated with left

    ventricular ectopy is thus similar to that which occurs in _____   *right*
    bundle branch block.

    The predominant forces travel from left to right *(away from/*
    toward) Lead V$_1$ and across the ventricular muscle tissue resulting   *toward*
    in a *(positive/negative)* and *(wide/narrow)* complex in this lead.   *positive*   *wide*

LV ECTOPY

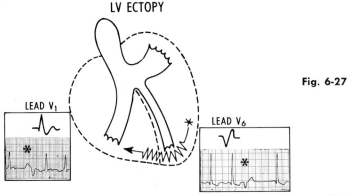

Fig. 6-27

135

92 We suggest monitoring on Lead V_1 to determine the origin of ventricular ectopy. In the setting of acute MI, most ventricular ectopic
beats originate from the left ventricle because this is the ventricle
most commonly injured. If ventricular ectopic beats are originating
in the right ventricle, they may also be the result of injury but
more likely they result from another mechanism, such as catheter
irritation of the ventricular wall.

Fascicular ectopy

93 Recent studies have proved that at times ventricular ectopic beats
may result in QRS complexes with only minimal widening. These
studies have shown that these "narrow PVCs" may originate in the
fascicles.
Remember: The LBB has two fascicles—the _____   *anterosuperior*

fascicle and the _____ fascicle.   *posteroinferior*

94 When ectopy originates in the divisions or fascicles, the QRS configuration will resemble the patterns associated with a *hemiblock.*
Remember: Hemiblocks are diagnosed by shifts in the electrical

_____, and they produce changes in the QRS morphology in Leads   *axis*

_____, _____, and aVF.   *I   II*
Thus Leads I, II, and aVF are also used in the diagnosis of fascicular ectopy.

Ectopy originating in the anterosuperior fascicle

95 *Let us review:* When an impulse is blocked in the posteroinferior
fascicle (LPH), there is *(RAD/ALAD).*   *RAD*
Lead I becomes *(negative/positive)* with an rS morphology, and   *negative*
Lead aVF becomes positive with a qR pattern.

96 When a ventricular ectopic beat originates in the anterosuperior
fascicle, the impulse activates the left ventricular muscle without
first activating the posterior fascicle. The posterior fascicle is not
physiologically blocked, but activation occurs in such a way that
this pathway is not used. Thus the pattern associated with anterior fascicular ectopy is the same as that which occurs in left

_____ hemiblock.   *posterior*
There is RAD associated with the ectopy because the forces travel
inferiorly and to the right *(away from/toward)* Lead I and *(away*   *away from*
from/toward) Lead aVF.   *toward*

97
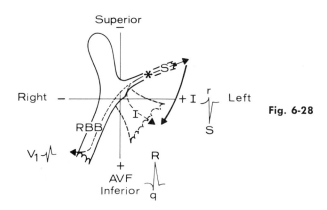
Fig. 6-28

Note: The anatomic relationship of the anterior fascicle to the right bundle branch is such that ectopic beats that arise in the anterior fascicle may not be delayed in their activation of the right ventricle.

Posterior fascicular ectopy

98 *Let us review:* When an impulse is blocked in the anterosuperior fascicle (LAH), there is *(RAD/ALAD)*.   *ALAD*
Lead I is predominantly *(positive/negative)* with a qR pattern and   *positive*
Leads II and aVF become *(positive/negative)* with an rS pattern.   *negative*

99 When a ventricular ectopic beat originates in the posteroinferior fascicle, the impulse activates the left ventricular muscle without first activating the anterior fascicle.
The anterior fascicle is not physiologically blocked, but activation occurs in such a way that this pathway is not used. Thus the pattern associated with posterior fascicular ectopy is the same as that

which occurs in left _____ hemiblock. There is ALAD asso-   *anterior*
ciated with the ectopy because the forces travel superiorly and to
the left *(away from/toward)* Lead I and *(away from/toward)* Lead   *toward*   *away from*
aVF.

100

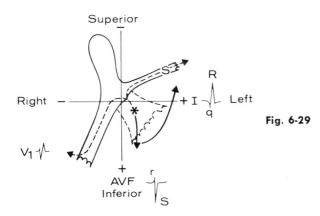

Fig. 6-29

Note: The anatomic relationship of the posterior fascicle to the RBB is such that if impulses arise in this fascicle there is usually some associated degree of RBBB.

101 PVCs with narrow QRS complexes have the same potential for producing repetitive ventricular firing or cardiac arrest when falling during the vulnerable period of a preceding beat as the usual PVC with a wide QRS complex.

Suggested readings

Castellanos, A., and Lemberg, L.: A programmed introduction to the electrical axis and action potential, 1974, Tampa Tracings.
Castellanos, A., and Lemberg, L.: Diagnosis of isolated and combined block in the bundle branches and the divisions of the left branch, Circulation 40:111, 1971.
Castellanos, A., and others: Post-infarction conduction disturbances; a self-teaching program, Dis. Chest 56:421, 1969.
Castellanos, A., and others: Alternating and co-existing block in the divisions of the left bundle branch, Dis. Chest 56:104, 1969.
Castellanos, A., Spence, M. I., and Chapell, D.: A nursing approach; hemiblocks and bundle branch blocks, Heart Lung 1:Jan.-Feb., 1972.
Damato, A. N., and Lau, S. H.: Clinical value of the electrogram of the conduction system, Prog. Cardiov. Dis. 13:119, 1970.
Dubin, D.: Rapid interpretation of EKG's, Tampa, Fla., 1970, Cover Publishing Co.
Gould, S. E., editor: Pathology of the heart,

Springfield, Ill., 1968, Charles C Thomas, Publisher.

Julian, D. G., and others: Prolongation of QRS duration in acute myocardial infarction, Prog. Cardiov. Dis. 13:56, 1970.

Mariott, H. T. L.: Practical electrocardiography, Baltimore, 1968, The Williams & Wilkins Co.

Pryor, R., and Blount, S. G.: The clinical significance of true L axis deviation, Am. Heart J. 72:391, 1966.

Rosenbaum, M. B.: Intraventricular trifascicular block, Heart Lung 1(2):216, Mar.-Apr. 1972.

Rosenbaum, M., Elizari, M. V., and Lazzari, J. O.: The hemiblocks, Oldsman, Fla., 1970, Tampa Tracings.

Rothfield, E. L., and others: The electrocardiographic syndrome of superior axis and right bundle branch block, Dis. Chest 55:306, 1969.

Scanlon, P. J., Pryor, R., and Blount, G.: Right bundle branch block associated with left superior and inferior intraventricular block, Circulation 42:1123, 1970.

Schamroth, L.: An introduction to electrocardiography, Edinburgh, 1971, Blackwell Scientific Publications.

Mechanical complications in acute myocardial infarction—heart failure and shock

HEART FAILURE

1 In previous units we have discussed normal and abnormal electrical activity in the heart.
Let us now consider the mechanical activity of the heart, or its role

as a _____.   *pump*

2 The function of the heart is to provide an adequate *supply of*

_____ *blood* to meet the metabolic *demands* of the   *oxygenated*
body's tissues.

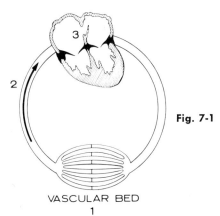

Fig. 7-1

VASCULAR BED
1

3 The function of the heart as a pump depends on three main factors:

(1) resistance to ejection of blood *(peripheral vascular* _____*)*;   *resistance*
(2) venous return to the heart, which is related to total *blood*

_____; and (3) contractility of the heart _____.   *volume*   *muscle*
The peripheral vascular resistance is also known as the heart's *af-*
terload. The venous return is also known as the heart's *preload.*
Disturbances in any of these variables may cause mechanical dysfunction of the heart and result in a discrepancy between the

_____ of blood and the _____ of the body's tissue.   *supply*   *demands*
The heart then may *fail* in its function as a pump. This condition is

known as heart _____.   *failure*

4 If the heart must pump blood against increased *vascular resistance*

or _____load, heart _____ may occur.   *after-*   *failure*
Remember: Vascular resistance is a major determinant of blood

_____. Systemic hypertension, then, is an example of a   *pressure*
(volume/pressure) load.   *pressure*

5 If the heart is presented with excessive volume or a _____load that   *pre*

it is unable to pump _____ _____ may occur. Administration   *heart failure*
of large amounts of intravenous fluids is an example of a *(volume/*   *volume*
pressure) load. Fluid overload is, thus, a potential source of heart
failure in patients with borderline cardiac reserve.

6 If the heart *muscle*, or *myocardium*, is damaged, _____ _____   *heart failure*
may occur. In the setting of acute MI, the myocardium *(is/is not)*   *is*
damaged.
It can then be expected that in acute MI some manifestations of

_____ _____ will be seen.   *heart failure*
Remember: Most myocardial infarctions predominantly involve the
(right/left) ventricle. Therefore, heart failure in the setting of   *left*
myocardial infarction is usually *(right/left)* sided heart failure.   *left*

7 When the heart fails to pump enough blood forward, some blood
becomes "dammed up." This produces congestion in the heart and
blood vessels draining into the heart. The patient will develop symptoms due to this *congestion*. Heart failure is thus frequently re-

ferred to as _____ heart failure, or *CHF*.   *congestive*

8 When the heart fails to pump enough blood forward, *cardiac output*
falls. The patient may therefore also exhibit symptoms of decreased

_____ _____.   *cardiac output*
The patient in heart failure, then, may exhibit symptoms due to:
(1) _____ or (2) decreased _____ _____.   *congestion; cardiac*
        output
9 The right and left side of the heart may fail together or *separately*.

We therefore speak of *right* ventricular failure or _____ ventricular   *left*
failure.
Heart failure in the setting of acute MI is usually *(right/left)* ven-   *left*
tricular failure.

Left ventricular failure

10 When the *left ventricle* is damaged, the heart cannot function effi-

ciently as a(n) _____. As a result, blood is "dammed up" behind   *pump*

the _____ _____. This produces congestion and increased   *left ventricle*

pressure in the left side of the heart and the _____ _____   *blood vessels*

draining into the _____ side of the heart.   *left*

11 Failure of the left ventricle, then, results in an *(increase/decrease)*   *increase*

in pressure, which is transmitted retrogradely to the left _____,   *atrium*

the pulmonary_____, and the pulmonary capillaries.   *veins*
This increase in pulmonary capillary pressure and pulmonary congestion causes fluid to escape from the alveolar capillaries into the

interstitial spaces of the _____.   *lungs*

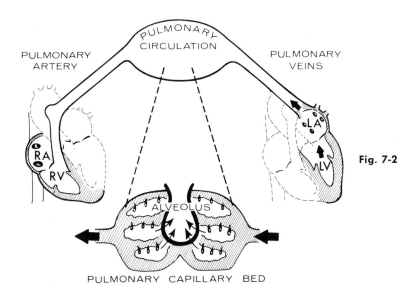

PULMONARY CIRCULATION

PULMONARY ARTERY

PULMONARY VEINS

Fig. 7-2

ALVEOLUS

PULMONARY CAPILLARY BED

12 Left heart failure may result in congestion of blood in the

_____ vascular bed. This could result in transudation of fluid   *pulmonary*
into the lungs.
Initially, fluid transudates into the *interstitial* spaces of the lungs.
When fluid is in the interstitial spaces, this state is known as
(interstitial/intracellular) edema.   *interstitial*
Fluid may then move into the *alveoli*. The presence of fluid in the

alveoli is known *clinically* as _____ edema.   *pulmonary*

13 The *pulmonary congestion* may be manifested by certain symptoms:
(1) dyspnea and cough, (2) orthopnea, (3) rales or wheezes, and
(4) frothy bloody sputum (hemoptysis).

14 *Dyspnea* is a subjective sensation of difficulty in breathing. In this
setting this symptom is directly related to an *(increase/decrease)*   *increase*
in pulmonary pressure secondary to *(left/right)* heart failure. The   *left*
resulting pulmonary congestion causes the lungs to become stiff
and less compliant. The effect is a(n) *(increase/decrease)* in the   *increase*

work of breathing, manifested symptomatically as _____.   *dyspnea*
Cough is another symptom of *(right/left)* heart failure and fre-   *left*
quently accompanies dyspnea.

15 The symptoms of dyspnea are related to position. *Orthopnea* implies
that a patient with stiff, congested lungs has greater dyspnea when

in the recumbent position and less dyspnea when in the _____   *upright*
position. In the upright position, venous return is decreased, hydro-
static pressure is decreased, and lung capacity is increased.

16 Auscultation of the lungs in the patient with heart failure may re-
veal *abnormal breath sounds*. The movement of air through abnormal *fluid* in the terminal air passages or alveoli produces a noise
known as a *rale*.
The *quality* of the rales is dependent upon their *origin*. The movement of air into fluid-filled *alveoli* produces fine crackling sounds.
These rales are heard best at the *end of inspiration* and do not dis-

141

appear with coughing. Fine end inspiratory rales indicate fluid in

the _____ or, mild _____ ventricular heart failure.　　　　*alveoli*　*left*

17 The rales of heart failure may be heard bilaterally or unilaterally on
the *right side.*
Note: Early left heart failure may be detected on chest x-ray as

pulmonary venous engorgement, *before* _____ may be heard at　*rales*
the bedside.

Severe pulmonary edema

18 The movement of air through fluid in the *bronchial (larger)* passages produces rales with a coarser, bubbling quality. These rales
are heard during expiration as well as during inspiration.

Coarse, bubbling rales indicate fluid in the _____　*bronchial*

_____, or severe _____ ventricular heart failure.　　*passages*　*left*

19 The movement of air through obstructed bronchioles *during expiration* produces a sound known as a *wheeze.* In severe pulmonary congestion, airway walls may become edematous and therefore narrowed. Air movement will meet an obstruction and result in a

_____.　　　　　　　　　　　　　　　　　　　　　*wheeze*

Another symptom in severe heart failure is *pink,* frothy sputum. It
results from the mixture of fluid, red cells, and air within the al-

veoli and is indicative of severe _____ edema.　　　*pulmonary*

20 Patients with left heart failure may also manifest symptoms of de-

creased _____ _____. When cardiac output falls, a se-　*cardiac output*
ries of compensatory mechanisms is initiated in order to maintain
an adequate blood supply to the heart and brain. (See Unit 3.)

The most important mechanisms are: (1) _____ heart rate　*increased*

(*Remember:* Cardiac output = stroke volume × _____　*ventricular*

_____.) and (2) *constriction* of blood vessels to the *skin, kidney,*　*rate*
and abdominal viscera.

21 The symptoms of decreased *cardiac output* include:

— heart—_____ heart _____　　　　　　　　*increased*　*rate*
— kidneys—decreased urinary output or oliguria
— skin—dusky, cool, moist
— brain—lethargy, dizziness, confusion, agitation
The fall in cardiac output and the vasoconstriction of the vessels to

the kidneys causes _____ renal perfusion, which results　*decreased*

in _____ urinary output, or _____.　　　　*decreased*　*oliguria*
A fall in cardiac output will also trigger compensatory mechanisms,

which will result in changes in _____ color and temperature.　*skin*
The skin assumes a dusky color from extraction of oxygen from
the capillaries. Skin temperature falls when blood is shunted from
the skin to more critical tissues.
A decrease in cardiac output to the brain results in *(increased/
decreased)* cerebral perfusion. Decreased perfusion to the brain is　*decreased*

manifested by *sensorium changes* such as lethargy, dizziness, confusion, and agitation.

Sensorium changes are usually a sign of severely _____ cardiac output and, therefore, might accompany the onset of

_____ heart failure.

decreased

severe

22 *Let us review:*

The two main problems associated with *left* heart failure are:

1. _____ congestion

pulmonary

2. *low* _____ _____

The clinical symptoms of pulmonary congestion include:

cardiac output

1. _____ and _____

dyspnea   orthopnea

2. _____

cough

3. _____ and/or _____

rales   wheezes

4. _____ and/or _____ _____

The organs affected by a decrease in cardiac output include the

frothy; bloody sputum

_____, _____, _____, and _____.

Symptoms related to a fall in cardiac output are:

heart; kidney; skin; brain

1. increased _____ _____

heart rate

2. decreased urine output, or _____

oliguria

3. changes in skin _____ and _____

color   temperature

4. change in _____

Left ventricular failure causes an increase in left _____ pressure,

sensorium

atrial

which is transmitted retrogradely to the _____ veins and capillaries. An increase in pulmonary capillary pressure may then be transmitted retrogradely to the pulmonary *(artery/vein)* and the *(right/left)* ventricle.

pulmonary

artery

right

This overloads the right ventricle and may cause _____ of the *right ventricle.*

failure

Note: The most common cause of right ventricular failure is _____

_____ failure.

left

ventricular

Right ventricular failure

23 The earliest sign of right sided failure is an increased right atrial (RA) pressure.

Right atrial pressure is also called *central venous pressure.* A catheter may be placed in the right atrium and the pressure measured against a column of water. This measurement is called the

_____ _____ _____ measurement, or CVP.

central venous pressure

24 An increase in CVP indicates an increase in pressure in the *(right/left)* side of the heart.

right

An increased CVP, therefore, reflects *(right/left)* heart failure.

right

An increased CVP *may indirectly* reflect left ventricular failure; however, an increased CVP *(does/does not) always* reflect left ventricular failure.

does not

Remember: The most common cause of right sided failure is _____

left

sided failure. Therefore, an increased CVP may indirectly reflect

_____ _____ _____.   *left ventricular failure*

25 An increase in the CVP can be observed clinically by distention of the *neck veins*, which feed into the superior vena cava and the

_____ atrium.   *right*

Congestion in the right side of the heart may progress beyond the right atrium into the *(venous/arterial)* side of the systemic circula-   *venous*
tion. Just as pulmonary edema is a symptom of left heart failure,

systemic edema is a manifestation of _____ heart failure.   *right*

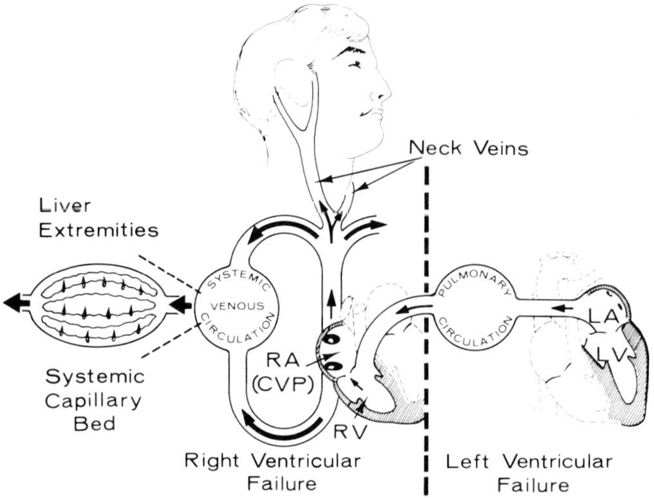

Fig. 7-3

26 The problem of systemic congestion may be manifested by certain symptoms: (1) liver enlargement and (2) peripheral edema.
The *liver* may become enlarged as a result of chronic, passive con-

gestion related to _____ _____.   *heart failure*
The development of *peripheral edema*, a late sign of _____   *heart*

_____, is best seen in the dependent parts of the body, usu-   *failure*
ally the feet and ankles.
Note: Patients with chronic left ventricular failure may develop right ventricular failure over a period of time. However, in the setting of acute MI, it is *uncommon* to see the symptoms of *(left/right)* heart failure.   *right*

27 *Let us review:* The most common cause of right heart failure is

_____ heart failure.   *left*
One of the earliest signs of right heart failure is an increase in *(LA/RA)* pressure. Changes in the right atrial pressure may be   *RA*

demonstrated by changes in the measurement of the _____. The   *CVP*

failure of the right side of the heart may result in _____   *systemic*
congestion.

28 The patient in heart failure may exhibit symptoms related to: (1)
                                                                  cardiac output;
low _____ _____ and (2) congestion—_____   *pulmonary*

and/or _____.   *systemic*

In most settings the *decreased cardiac output* and *congestion* have a *common* underlying mechanism: *decreased myocardial contractility*. Therefore, initial therapy in the management of heart failure in acute MI is directed toward *decreasing* the *workload,* or the demand, on the weakened myocardium.

This may be accomplished by: (1) promoting physical and psychological rest and (2) providing supplementary oxygen.

29 Therapy may also be directed toward *improving myocardial contractility.*

The most commonly used drug for this purpose is digitalis. Digitalis increases myocardial _____ and thus *(increases/ decreases)* the pulmonary and systemic congestion.

contractility
decreases

30 Pulmonary and systemic congestion may also be decreased by *decreasing circulating blood volume* and *interstitial fluids*. This may be accomplished by administering *diuretics* and by *restriction of sodium (Na⁺) intake.*

Therapy directed toward decreasing pulmonary and systemic congestion usually consists of decreasing *circulating* _____

blood

_____ by: administering _____ and restricting _____ intake.

volume; diuretics; Na^+

31 *Pulmonary* congestion and edema may be *rapidly* corrected by *decreasing the venous return* to the heart and lungs. This mode of therapy is indicated in life-threatening settings.

Reduction of the venous return to the heart may be accomplished by placing the patient in Fowler's position and by the application of *rotating tourniquets,* which trap blood in the extremities. *Morphine* acts as a vasodilator and thereby *(increases/decreases)* venous return to the heart. The administration of *intermittent positive pressure* ventilation can also serve to *mechanically* decrease venous return to the heart. Alcohol may be added as a defoaming agent.

decreases

IN SUMMARY:

32 The patient in heart failure may exhibit symptoms related to: (1) low _____ _____ and (2) congestion—_____

cardiac output;
pulmonary

and/or _____.

systemic

Four main principles are employed in the management of these problems.

To increase cardiac output and decrease congestion:

— decrease cardiac _____

workload

— strengthen the _____

myocardium

To decrease pulmonary and systemic congestion:

— decrease circulating _____ _____

blood volume

To decrease pulmonary congestion:

— decrease _____ _____

venous return

33 Let us briefly consider the specific problem of *acute pulmonary edema* or severe *pulmonary congestion.*

Acute pulmonary edema is seen most frequently in the presence of *(right/left)* ventricular failure.

left

Remember: Pulmonary congestion may be manifested by these symptoms:

1. _____ or _____   *dyspnea   cough*

2. _____   *orthopnea*

3. _____ and _____   *rales   wheezes*

4. _____   *hemoptysis*

Note: Pulmonary congestion in *acute* pulmonary edema is severe and the symptoms are dramatic. All of the above symptoms are present.

34 The management of acute pulmonary edema consists of these therapeutic measures. The administration of *morphine sulfate* is important in this therapy. It acts directly by dilating peripheral veins, thus causing a(n) *(increase/decrease)* in venous return. Morphine   *decrease* also decreases pulmonary venous pressure. Other desirable effects of morphine adminstration are a reduction in both anxiety and

_____ rate.   *respiratory*

Morphine acts as a *(vasodilator/vasoconstrictor)* and thus decreases   *vasodilator*

_____ _____ to the heart. Therefore, the patient must be   *venous return*

monitored for depression of blood _____.   *pressure*

Morphine also depresses respirations. Therefore, the nurse must

observe for _____ depression.   *respiratory*

35 *Diuretic agents* may be used to *(decrease/increase)* blood volume   *decrease* and pulmonary congestion. Most of the major diuretics in common

use act by blocking the reabsorption of _____ and _____ in the Na^+ *water* kidneys.

36 Aminophylline acts mainly in the lungs as a vasodilator and bronchodilator. It therefore may be given to *(increase/decrease)* pulmo-   *decrease* nary venous pressure. It has an effect on the heart of increasing myocardial contractility. A diuretic response occurs in the kidney.

37 *Nursing orders:* Drug therapy
   1. Anticipate and prepare for the administration of morphine sulfate, aminophylline, and diuretic agents.
   2. When administering morphine sulfate the nurse should watch for

   _____ and _____ _____ depression.   *respiratory; blood pressure*
   3. When administering aminophylline, the nurse should watch for nausea, vomiting, sinus tachycardia, and ventricular arrhythmias.
   4. When administering diuretic agents, the nurse should record the

   diuretic response and watch for fluid and _____ deple-   *electrolyte* tion.

38 Rotating tourniquets may be applied to *(increase/decrease)* venous   *decrease* return to the heart. The action is to trap blood in the large muscle masses of the extremities. *Note:* The use of rotating tourniquets is contraindicated in the presence of hypotension, because they cause

a decrease in _____ _____ to the heart.   *venous return*

Nursing orders: Rotating tourniquets

1. Place tourniquets in a position high in groin and axilla.
2. Check blood pressure before and during use of the tourniquets; rotating tourniquets are contraindicated if the patient is *(hypo-/ hyper-)*tensive.   *hypo-*
3. Check for the presence and adequacy of arterial pulses—only the venous flow should be occluded.
4. Occlude only three extremities at one time; rotate at least every 10 to 15 minutes.
5. When discontinuing tourniquets, do *not* release all at one time.

39 Supplementary oxygen may be given to increase arterial oxygen saturation.
The administration of intermittent positive pressure breathing (IPPB) may be used to cause a decrease in central blood volume by

decreasing _____ return. This therapy may also enhance pul-   *venous*
monary ventilation in patients with a low Po_2 and high CO_2 levels.
Nursing orders: Oxygen therapy
1. In patients who are "mouth breathers" or are hyperventilating, a mask may be the preferable means of oxygen administration.
2. Administer low flow rates of oxygen to patients with a history of chronic CO_2 retention and a hypoxic respiratory drive.
3. If administering IPPB therapy, watch for patient fatigue and hypotension, increases in heart rate, and/or the appearance of rhythm disturbances.
4. Antifoaming agents such as alcohol may be administered by IPPB to facilitate removal of edema fluid.
5. Evaluate respiratory status by auscultating the lung fields, observing character of respirations, and assessing arterial blood gases.
6. Document effectiveness of oxygen therapy on blood gases. (See Unit 3.)

40 Patients with acute pulmonary edema are in acute respiratory distress and are experiencing apprehension. Nursing measures to promote patient comfort and relieve anxiety are indicated.
Nursing orders: Acute pulmonary edema
1. Help patient to assume comfortable position—trunk should be upright and legs dependent (downward); some patients are most comfortable at chair rest.
2. Explain frightening procedures carefully (tourniquets, IPPB therapy, phlebotomy).
3. Relieve needs for oxygen or analgesics promptly, thereby decreasing anxiety.
4. Provide an atmosphere that is conducive to rest.

IN SUMMARY:
Nursing orders: Heart failure
1. Provide cardiac rest
   — place patient in semi-Fowler's or Fowler's position
   — encourage chair rest
   — allow use of commode chair
   — relieve psychological stress
      — explain all procedures in simple terms
      — allow contact with familiar objects
      — encourage independence and self-care
      — allow visitors with limitations as needed
   — administer sedation as required

2. Observe patient for overt signs of dyspnea
   — shortness of breath
   — cough
   — increase in respiratory rale
   — Valsalva respirations
3. Auscultate the heart and lungs when checking vital signs; check for:
   — gallops ⎫
             ⎬ See Unit 7, frames 88-118
   — murmurs ⎭
   — variations in the normal heart sounds
   — rales
   — alterations in the quality of the normal breath sounds
4. Check the CVP when checking vital signs
   — if no CVP catheter is inserted, observe for the development of neck vein distention
   — always correlate CVP findings with lung sounds
5. Watch for the development of signs of decreased cardiac output
6. In the presence of *pulmonary edema*
   — place patient in high Fowler's position
   — turn down intravenous fluids to keep line open
   — start oxygen
   — obtain vital signs
   — have available at bedside
     — rotating tourniquets
     — IPPB equipment
     — resuscitation equipment
     — morphine sulfate
     — aminophylline
     — diuretics
     — digitalis

HEMODYNAMIC CHANGES IN ACUTE MI

41 In the setting of acute MI, the myocardial damage and resulting mechanical dysfunction alter the movement of blood through the heart. The study and/or monitoring of these alterations in the movement of blood is known as *hemodynamics*.

42 *Let us review:* The major mechanical events of the heart are ventricular systole and ventricular _____.   *diastole*
Systole refers to the ejecting period of the ventricles. Diastole refers to the _____ period.   *filling*

43 The first change occurring in a damaged myocardium affects *diastole.*
Remember: Myocardial infarction involves predominantly *(right/ left)* ventricular muscle. Therefore, the first mechanical changes   *left*
that occur in acute MI affect *left ventricular (systole/diastole).*   *diastole*

44 Like the tissue of the lungs, myocardial tissue has the ability to stretch. This ability of the myocardium to stretch with entering volume is known as *compliance*. The first sign of left ventricular dysfunction in acute MI is a decrease in compliance in the affected area.
As the ventricles become less compliant, they become more resistant to stretch. Ventricles thus affected have difficulty accepting entering blood volume, and the ventricular *diastolic* pressure rises.

148

45 *Let us review:* The first mechanical changes that occur in acute MI
affect left ventricular *(systole/diastole)*. The first sign of left ventricular dysfunction in acute MI is a rise in left ventricular   *diastole*

_____ pressure, caused by alterations in _____.   *diastolic; compliance*

46 Left ventricular filling occurs in two phases. The *first* filling phase
occurs as the A-V valves open at the onset of diastole. The *second*
phase occurs at the end of diastole as atrial contraction completes
ventricular filling.

47 A slightly damaged left ventricle can accommodate the blood that
enters during the *initial* filling phase. However, because of alterations in compliance, the left ventricle cannot efficiently accommodate the *added* volume that enters with atrial contraction.
Remember: Atrial contraction occurs at the *(beginning/end)* of   *end*
ventricular diastole. Thus left ventricular pressure first rises at the
end of diastole.
The first hemodynamic change seen as a result of acute MI is—

more accurately—a rise in left ventricular _____ diastolic pressure   *end*
(LVEDP).

48 The second change in mechanical function affects ventricular *sys-*
tole resulting in a fall in cardiac output.
In the initial stages of myocardial damage, the *unaffected* fibers
may increase their contractility and overcompensate for the loss of
effective contractile structures. Thus there is no initial net loss in
contractility, and the cardiac output is maintained.

49 Subsequent loss of myocardial function results in the inability of
the intact fibers to compensate for this loss. The cardiac output
therefore falls.
When the cardiac output falls as a result of mechanical dysfunction
and the demands of the tissues are no longer effectively met, the
heart has failed to perform as an effective pump. This state is now
known as *heart failure.*
Note: Mechanical dysfunction is assumed to be the mechanism of
the fall in cardiac output when inadequate volume, rhythm, or peripheral resistance has been ruled out as a causative factor.

50 *Let us review:* The second hemodynamic change occurring in acute

MI is a fall in _____ _____.   *cardiac output*
A fall in cardiac output due to mechanical dysfunction is known as

_____ _____.   *heart failure*

51 Following acute MI and usually accompanying the fall in cardiac
output, the injured left ventricle *may* not completely eject its contents during systole. As a result, residual volume remains in the
left ventricle at the end of systole and the beginning of diastole.
At the onset of diastole the left ventricle is already partially full
and has difficulty accepting even the initial amounts of entering
blood. Thus, even initially, the diastolic pressure *(increases/de-*   *increases*
creases).

52 *Remember:* During *ventricular diastole* the valves separating the
left atrium from the left ventricle are *(open/closed)*. The left atrial   *open*
and left ventricular chambers thus communicate with each other,
and the rise in the left ventricular pressure is transmitted to the

149

left atrium (LA). This increase in pressure is further transmitted

retrogradely to the communicating pulmonary _____ and pulmo-   *veins*

nary _____ resulting in *pulmonary congestion*. (See Fig.   *capillaries*
7-2, frames 10 to 17.)
The third hemodynamic change occurring in acute MI is *pulmonary congestion* caused by a further rise in LVEDP.

IN SUMMARY:

53 The three progressive hemodynamic changes that may occur as a
    result of acute MI are:
    1. a rise in left ventricular _____ diastolic pressure (LVEDP) due   *end*

       to altered _____   *compliance*

    2. a fall in the _____ _____   *cardiac output*

    3. _____ _____ due to a further rise in LV dias-   *pulmonary congestion*
       tolic pressure

54 When considering the disturbances in myocardial function that
    occur in the setting of acute MI, the factors affecting myocardial
    oxygen consumption must also be evaluated. The determinants of
    myocardial oxygen consumption (MVO_2) are:
    1. heart *rate*
    2. heart *radius*, which influences the wall tension (as determined by
       the volume of filling, or *preload*)
    3. the *pressure* load (as determined by the peripheral vascular re-
       sistance, or *afterload*)
    4. myocardial *contractility*
    In the setting of acute MI, myocardial injury may extend resulting
    in further dysfunction if the discrepancy between myocardial oxy-
    gen supply and demand is magnified.
    Therefore, prophylactic action should be taken to minimize myo-
    cardial oxygen demands and to improve the coronary blood supply.
    (See Nursing orders for hemodynamic monitoring, frame 86 and
    shock, frame 157.)

HEMODYNAMIC MONITORING

55 The major hemodynamic alterations in acute MI involve changes
    in left ventricular *pressure* and *ejection* (the cardiac output).
    Therefore, the monitoring of hemodynamic changes should include

    attempts at monitoring left ventricular _____ directly or indi-   *pressure*

    rectly and monitoring changes in the _____ _____.   *cardiac output*

56 This monitoring may be done either invasively or noninvasively.
    Noninvasive evaluation includes monitoring of heart sounds and
    detection of clinical signs of pulmonary congestion and decreased
    cardiac output mentioned earlier in this unit. (See frame 22.)
    Another currently used noninvasive method of evaluationg left ven-
    tricular function (both systolic and diastolic) is *echocardiography*.
    A beam of sound is directed through the patient's chest wall from
    anterior to the posterior.
    The beam bounces back vibrating, or echoing, when it makes con-
    tact with any dense structure such as the ventricular wall or valves.
    The pattern of these vibrations is recorded and provides informa-
    tion about the function of the mechanical structures.

57 At the present time noninvasive techniques of hemodynamic monitoring have not provided as practical, accurate, or as early information about left ventricular pressure and output as the invasive modes.

The advent of the Swan-Ganz flow-directed balloon-tipped catheter has popularized the use of invasive techniques at the bedside.

MONITORING PRESSURES (INVASIVE TECHNIQUES)

58 *Let us review:* The first mechanical changes occurring in acute MI affect *left ventricular (systolic/diastolic)* pressure. Left ventricular pressure rises first at the *(beginning/end)* of diastole.

diastolic

end

Therefore, the goal of monitoring pressure changes in acute MI is

to detect as accurately as possible early changes in _____ _____

left ventricular

_____ _____ _____ (LVEDP).

end diastolic pressure

59 The most accurate measure of LVEDP is obtained directly via a left ventricular catheter.

60 However, since the right side of the heart is more easily accessible via the venous system, indirect monitoring of left ventricular changes is done via catheters introduced into the right side of the heart.

61 *Early* attempts to monitor left ventricular function were done through catheters introduced into the right atrium recording the

_____ _____ pressure.

central venous

However, the right atrium communicates with the *(right ventricle/ left ventricle)* only during ventricular diastole and thus reflects changes only in *(RVEDP/LVEDP)*.

right ventricle

RVEDP

62 Pressures recorded from the pulmonary artery were found to correlate more closely with left ventricular function because the pulmonary artery is obviously anatomically closer to the left ventricular cavity than are the right atrium and right ventricle.

In addition, the catheter is situated beyond the pulmonary valve. Closure of the pulmonary valve during ventricular diastole interrupts communication with the *(right/left)* side of the heart.

right

However, direct communication is maintained with the pulmonary circulation and the *(right/left)* atrium. (See Fig. 7-4, p. 152.)

left

Since the left atrium, in turn, communicates with the left ventricle during diastole, communication is established between the pulmonary artery and left ventricle.

Thus pulmonary artery end diastolic pressure closely approximates

the pressure in the _____ circulation, and, in the absence

pulmonary

of pulmonary hypertension, _____ atrial pressure and _____.

left   LVEDP

Continuous monitoring of pulmonary artery pressure is made possible via a balloon-tipped flow-directed Swan-Ganz catheter.

63 Although the monitoring of pulmonary artery *(systolic/diastolic)* pressure in acute MI is a useful index of left ventricular function, a still more accurate measurement is obtainable.

diastolic

The balloon of the Swan-Ganz catheter can be deflated so that the catheter may be advanced further into one of the branches of the pulmonary artery.

64 Since in this position the catheter is closer to the pulmonary capil-

MONITORING OF VENTRICULAR DIASTOLIC PRESSURES

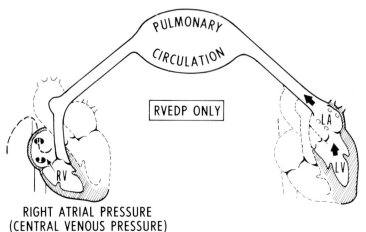

RVEDP ONLY

RIGHT ATRIAL PRESSURE
(CENTRAL VENOUS PRESSURE)

THE SWAN-GANZ CATHETER

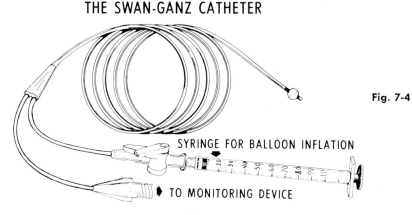

SYRINGE FOR BALLOON INFLATION

TO MONITORING DEVICE

Fig. 7-4

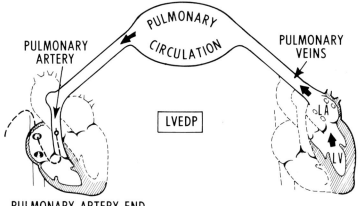

PULMONARY ARTERY

PULMONARY VEINS

LVEDP

PULMONARY ARTERY END
DIASTOLIC PRESSURE (PAEDP)

lary bed than it is in the main pulmonary artery, the pressure re-

cording obtained at this site is known as *pulmonary* _____ *capillary*
pressure.

When the catheter is in position, the balloon is inflated so that the
catheter becomes *wedged* in the vessel. The pressure obtained after

the catheter is wedged is known as the pulmonary capillary _____   *wedge*
pressure.

65 The wedging of the catheter in the pulmonary artery branch not
    only interrupts communication with the *(right/left)* side of the   *right*
    heart but also interrupts communication with part of the pulmo-
    nary circulation.
    Therefore, as compared with the pulmonary artery pressure, pul-
    monary capillary wedge pressure is a *(more/less)* accurate index of   *more*
    left atrial and left ventricular end diastolic function.

PULMONARY CAPILLARY WEDGE PRESSURE

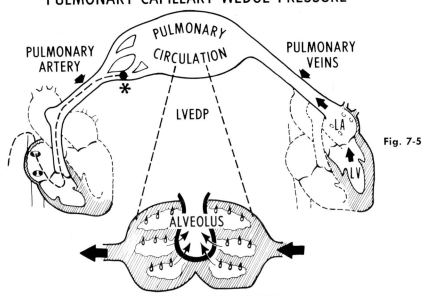

Fig. 7-5

66 The most common potential complications associated with the use
    of Swan-Ganz catheters are: (1) *right ventricular PVCs and ven-*
    tricular tachycardia resulting from mechanical stimulation of the
    ventricular wall during insertion and during monitoring if the
    catheter slips back into the right ventricle and (2) *pulmonary in-*
    farction caused by prolonged pulmonary ischemia if the catheter re-
    mains inflated in the wedge position.
    Note: The length of time the catheter is tolerated in the wedge po-
    sition is individually determined. However, prophylactically, wedge
    readings should be taken as quickly as possible and the balloon de-
    flated immediately until a pulmonary artery pulse pattern is again
    obtained.

67 Normally LVEDP is approximately 6 to 10 mm Hg. Elevations in
    LVEDP of approximately 12 to 15 mm Hg are expected in the set-
    ting of acute MI.
    Pulmonary artery end diastolic (PAEDP) and pulmonary capillary
    wedge pressures usually *(do/do not)* reflect LVEDP. Therefore,   *do*

    PAEDP and wedge pressure readings should not exceed _____ _____   *12 to*

    _____ mm Hg in acute MI.   *15*
    Increases in pressures beyond this level may indicate greater
    (right ventricular/left ventricular) dysfunction and predict impend- *left ventricular*

153

ing _____ congestion. Such changes indicate left ventric-   *pulmonary*

ular _____.   *failure*

68 A wedge pressure of 5 mg Hg would indicate a(n) *(increased/*
   decreased) LVEDP. The most likely explanation would be de-   *decreased*
   creased left ventricular filling because of blood volume depletion.
   Indicated therapy would consist of administering *(IV fluids/di-*   *IV fluids*
   uretics).

THE PRESSURE PULSE PATTERNS

69 Continuous monitoring of the pressure pulse patterns is necessary
   to: (1) effectively monitor catheter position and (2) record pressures accurately and thus avoid complications.
   Although pressure values may be recorded with a catheter-manom-
   eter system, a record of the pulse pattern can only be obtained with
   the use of a catheter-transducer system.

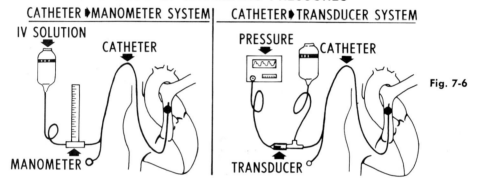

Fig. 7-6

70 With the use of a catheter-transducer system, characteristic patterns may be recorded from either *atria, ventricles,* or *arteries.*
   Recognition of these characteristic mechanical patterns has added
   a new dimension to the nursing management of critical care patients.

Ventricular patterns

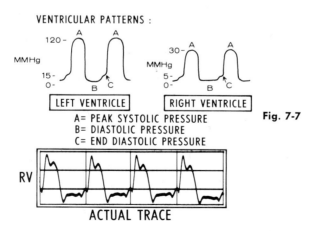

Fig. 7-7

71 Pressure within the right and left ventricle rises quickly with the
   onset of ventricular contraction, or *(systole/diastole)*. It rapidly   *systole*

reaches a peak point. This point is known as the peak _____   *systolic*
pressure.

As systolic ejection is completed, the *(A-V/semilunar)* valves close   *semilunar*

separating the ventricles from the _____ leaving them. The pres-   *vessels*

sure in the ventricles drops abruptly as ventricular filling, or

_____, begins.   *diastole*

The ventricular *end* diastolic pressure is recorded just before the
onset of the next systole.

Arterial patterns

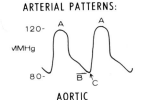

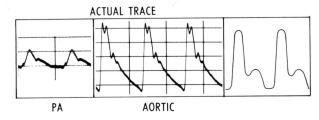

A= PEAK SYSTOLIC PRESSURE
B= LOWEST DIASTOLIC PRESSURE
C= END DIASTOLIC PRESSURE   **Fig. 7-8**

Note: Peripheral artery (brachial, femoral, or radial) may mimic
either of the two examples of aortic patterns above. The PA pattern
may also closely mimic the aortic or peripheral arterial pattern in
a given patient. (See frame 73.)

72 The pressure within the major arteries (pulmonary artery and
aorta) rises quickly as blood is ejected into them with the onset of

ventricular systole. It also rapidly reaches a peak _____   *systolic*
pressure.

Since the valves separating the ventricles and vessels are *(open/*   *open*
closed) during ventricular systole, ventricular systolic pressures
and arterial systolic pressures *(are/are not)* equivalent.   *are*

Arterial systolic pressure reflects the changes occurring within the

arteries during _____ systole.   *ventricular*

73 With the onset of ventricular diastole the semilunar valves *(open/*
close), separating the ventricles and the blood vessels.   *close*

The pressure in the vessels drops *gradually* as the blood still within
them is dispersed throughout the vascular bed to the tissues.

Remember: Ventricular diastolic pressure drops *(gradually/*
abruptly). Therefore, ventricular and arterial *systolic* patterns are   *abruptly*
similar, but their diastolic patterns are distinctly *(the same/differ-*   *different*
ent).

The record obtained from a catheter in a peripheral artery such as the *brachial* or *radial* artery may closely mimic the pulmonary artery or aortic patterns.

Atrial patterns (or pulmonary capillary wedge pattern)

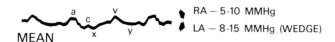

MEAN

> RA — 5-10 MMHg
> LA — 8-15 MMHg (WEDGE)

a = ATRIAL CONTRACTION
c = VENTRICULAR CONTRACTION
v = VENTRICULAR DIASTOLE
x & y = DROPS IN PRESSURE

ACTUAL TRACE

Fig. 7-9

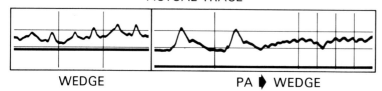

WEDGE   PA ▶ WEDGE

74 Pressures within the right and left atrium rise quickly with the onset of atrial contraction, producing an atrial systolic pulse wave recorded as the *a wave*.
The a wave in an atrial pulse pattern represents _____ _____.

atrial

contraction

75 Since the force of atrial contraction is not as great as the force of ventricular contraction, the atrial systolic pulse is not usually as distinctly noted on an oscilloscope record.
Ventricular mechanical events also directly influence atrial events, producing extra pulsations in the pressure pattern. (See Fig. 7-9.)
As a result, unlike ventricular and arterial patterns, the atrial pattern *(does/does not)* exhibit as distinct systolic and diastolic curves.
Instead, it assumes a wavy configuration. An average, or *mean,* pressure level is usually recorded.
Note: Since *pulmonary capillary wedge pressure* most directly reflects left atrial pressure, the characteristic wedge pulse pattern closely resembles the atrial pattern. (See Fig. 7-9, frames 63 to 65.)
Venous pulse patterns such as those present in the neck veins also resemble the atrial pattern because of their direct communication with the right atrium.

does not

MONITORING CARDIAC OUTPUT (INVASIVE TECHNIQUE)

76 Certain principles must be reviewed before the invasive techniques for monitoring cardiac output can be understood.
Remember: The purpose of maintaining effective cardiac output is to provide enough blood to the tissues to meet their _____ demands.
The demands of the tissues for oxygen (oxygen consumption needs), however, cannot be met by an adequate *blood supply* alone. The effective delivery of oxygen to the tissues is also dependent on the *oxygen content* of the blood.
Therefore: Tissue *demands* (oxygen consumption) = *blood supply* (cardiac output) × *oxygen supply* (oxygen content).

oxygen

156

77 The above principle is known as the *Fick principle*. This principle is used as a basis for calculating and clinically evaluating cardiac output.
Let us review: Oxygen delivery to the tissues may be affected by variations in:

   1. tissue _____ as occurs with increased metabolism — *demands*

   2. _____ _____ — *cardiac output*

   3. _____ _____ — *oxygen content*

78 When the cardiac output falls, the tissues must extract a greater amount of the oxygen content from each cc (ml) of blood in order to receive the same oxygen supply.
When there is evidence (on a blood gas analysis) that progressively greater amounts of oxygen are being extracted from the blood, a possible explanation is that the cardiac output is *(increasing/ decreasing)*. — *decreasing*

79 Subtraction of the oxygen content of a venous sample (returning from the tissues) from the oxygen content of an arterial sample (being delivered to the tissues) determines the content *extracted* by the tissues.
Tissue extraction of oxygen = arterial oxygen content − venous oxygen content.
Note: This difference in the oxygen content between arterial and venous blood is known as the *A-V oxygen difference*.
The amount of oxygen extracted from the blood by the tissues is

determined by calculating the _____ _____ difference. — *A-V oxygen*

80 *Let us review:* Calculation of the amount of oxygen extracted by

the tissues provides a basis for evaluating changes in _____ — *cardiac*

_____. — *output*

The amount of oxygen extracted is determined by comparing the

_____ _____ of arterial and venous samples. — *oxygen content*

81 The oxygen content of the blood is evaluated clinically by analysis

of the _____ and _____ _____ values obtained on a — *Po₂; oxygen saturation*
blood gas analysis. (See Unit 3.)
The oxygen saturation reflects the amount of oxygen _____ to — *bound*

hemoglobin. The Po_2 reflects the partial _____ exerted by — *pressure*
the smaller amounts of oxygen in solution, which are more freely available for immediate tissue use.

82 One method of determining cardiac output is to roughly estimate the A-V oxygen difference. The A-V oxygen difference may be estimated roughly by comparing the oxygen saturation values of a series of blood samples.
If the difference obtained in each set of samples becomes progressively greater, it is assumed that the cardiac output has *(increased/ decreased)*. — *decreased*
Remember: When the cardiac output falls, the tissues must remove

a greater amount of _____ from each cc of blood provided. — *oxygen*

83 A second method of determining cardiac output is by calculating the exact A-V oxygen difference.

The A-V oxygen difference may be calculated exactly by comparing the *total* oxygen content of arterial and venous samples—that which is dissolved as well as that bound to hemoglobin. This method

of calculation allows for a more accurate estimation of _____   *cardiac*

_____. *(Note formula:* O_2 content $= P_{O_2} \times 0.0003$ *plus*   *output*
$1.39 \times$ serum hemoglobin $\times$ percent O_2 *saturation.)*

84 The above methods of estimating cardiac output are based on the assumption that tissue consumption of oxygen remains stable.
A third method for determining cardiac output is by calculating tissue oxygen consumption. The amount of oxygen consumed by the tissues may be calculated with a special respirometer that measures the amount of oxygen inhaled and the amount exhaled by the patient.
When *both* tissue oxygen consumption and A-V oxygen difference are calculated, then a more *precise* determination of cardiac output can be obtained.
Remember:

   Tissue demands $=$ blood supply $\times$ oxygen supply extracted
(CO_2 consumption)   (CO)   (A-V O_2 difference)
Therefore:
Blood supply $=$ *oxygen consumption*
     (CO)   (_____ _____ _____)   *A-V oxygen difference*

85 A fourth method of determining cardiac output is by more sophisticated *indicator-dilution* techniques.

DYE DILUTION   THERMAL DILUTION

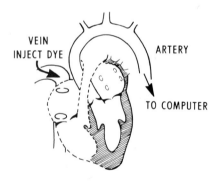
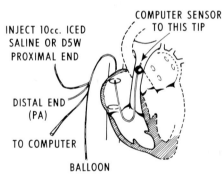

VEIN INJECT DYE   ARTERY   TO COMPUTER

INJECT 10cc. ICED SALINE OR D5W PROXIMAL END   COMPUTER SENSOR TO THIS TIP

DISTAL END (PA)   TO COMPUTER   BALLOON

Fig. 7-10

Note: A variation of the simple Swan-Ganz catheter is available with two additional lumens that allow for the monitoring of cardiac output by thermal dilution technique. The proximal lumen communicates with the right atrium when the distal tip is in the pulmo-

nary artery. Right atrial pressure, or the _____ _____   *central venous*

_____, may be monitored via this lumen. The thermistor lumen   *pressure*
communicates with the distal tip in the pulmonary artery and may be attached to a computer sensitive to temperature changes in the injected fluid, which will calculate the cardiac output.

86 *Nursing orders:* Hemodynamic monitoring
   1. While monitoring *pulmonary arterial* pressure, note characteristic pulmonary arterial pulse pattern on oscilloscope

— watch for changes in the pulse pattern that might indicate the catheter has slipped back into the right ventricle
— monitor on V_1 for right ventricular PVCs when catheter in right ventricle or during catheter insertion (see Unit 6); may inflate balloon to cushion tip
— keep xylocaine at bedside; may be given prophylactically during insertion or as per routine criteria
— record PAEDP if possible; with respiratory fluctuation, record on expiration
— note the presence or development of pulmonary complications that might invalidate correlations between PAEDP and LVEDP (increased pulmonary arterial systolic pressures may be a clue)
2. When obtaining pulmonary capillary *wedge* pressures:
— introduce only as much gas as required to obtain change from pulmonary artery to wedge pulse pattern on oscilloscope
— do not introduce more gas than is designated on balloon catheter
— record mean wedge pressure quickly, deflating balloon immediately thereafter; verify that catheter is no longer wedged by pattern change on scope (wedge back to pulmonary artery)
— if wedge pattern cannot be obtained with maximum inflation, notify physician and record PAEDP in the interim
3. While monitoring pressures invasively watch concurrently for noninvasive signs of increased LVEDP such as S_4 and especially S_3 gallop (See Auscultation of the heart, frames 88 to 118.)
— atrial arrhythmias
— signs of *pulmonary congestion* such as:
— increased respiratory rate, Valsalva (forced) respiration
— end-inspiratory rales not clearing with coughing
4. Institute nursing measures to maintain minimal oxygen demands by preventing and/or quickly correcting factors that might increase myocardial oxygen consumption (See nursing orders for shock, frame 159.)
5. Provide increased oxygen supply via supplementary oxygen; may document effectiveness on blood gases
6. Watch for further mechanical complications such as mitral insufficiency or VSD (ventricular septal defect) (murmurs) or aneurysm (with AWMI, palpable movement of chest wall)
7. Watch for intermittent changes in the pulse pattern that might indicate changes in contractility and cardiac output
— every other pressure pulse may be smaller in a patient with CHF as the heart cannot sustain strong pulses (pulsus alternans)
— with arrhythmias the pulse may become irregular and/or diminished as the output with these is less
— the voltage of the pattern may also vary with respiration due to respiratory influences on cardiac output
8. Give special care to catheter site for the prevention of endocarditis in the form of routine prep, dressing changes, and carefully sealed dressings; monitor temperature
9. Record serial changes in cardiac output; when evaluating the cardiac output results, relate them to the patient's body surface area *(cardiac index)*
10. As cardiac index begins to drop, monitor clinical signs of decreased tissue perfusion (noting a *symptomatic* fall in cardiac

output) that might indicate evolution of hemodynamics to the shock state

Note: For nursing action in the presence of significant elevations in LVEDP and significant decreases in LVEDP and cardiac output, refer to nursing orders for CHF, frame 40, and shock, frame 159.

AUSCULTATION OF THE HEART

87 *Remember:* The heart sounds serve as _____ outlining

    parameters

the _____ events of the heart.

    mechanical

Alterations in the mechanical activity of the heart are reflected by the presence of extra (sometimes abnormal) heart sounds and variations in the normal heart sounds.

88 *Let us review:* The earliest mechanical alterations occurring in an acute MI affect ventricular *(filling/contraction)*, which is also known as ventricular *(systole/diastole)*. Left ventricular pressure rises first at the *(beginning/end)* of diastole.

    filling
    diastole
    end

Variations in the heart sounds are produced that correlate with these changes in *(LAEDP/LVEDP)*. The heart sounds thus provide a means for clinically evaluating the *mechanical* and *hemodynamic* changes occurring in acute MI.

    LVEDP

89 The heart sounds are produced by the mechanical events that accompany valve closure.

S_1 marks the onset of ventricular *(systole/diastole)*.

    systole

During ventricular systole the *(A-V/semilunar)* valves close, the ventricular muscle wall contracts, and the blood is ejected into the

    A-V

_____ _____.

    blood vessels

Although older theories claim that valve closure is the major factor responsible for the production of the sound, more recent theories are less definite. The sound may be produced by any of *three* factors or a combination of them:

1. *valve closure*
2. vibrations of the ventricular wall associated with *ventricular contraction*
3. vibrations associated with *acceleration* and *deceleration* of blood by the force of ventricular contraction

90 S_2 marks the onset of ventricular *(systole/diastole)*.

    diastole

During ventricular diastole, the *(A-V/semilunar)* valves close, the ventricular wall relaxes, and blood enters the ventricles from the

    semilunar

_____.

    atria

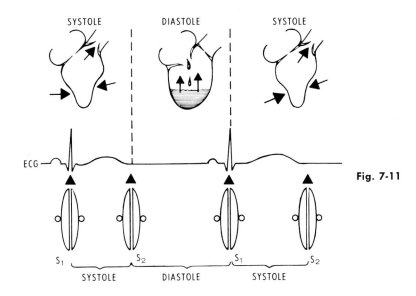

SYSTOLE   DIASTOLE   SYSTOLE

ECG

Fig. 7-11

S_1 S_2 S_1 S_2

SYSTOLE   DIASTOLE   SYSTOLE

Note: The electrical activity is presented to emphasize its relationship to the mechanical activity.

92   The most clinically significant abnormal heart sounds occurring in the setting of acute MI are *gallops* and *murmurs*.

The abnormal heart sounds that reflect left ventricular *diastolic* changes are the *gallops*.

Gallops

93   Gallops are extra sounds created by "gushes of blood" entering resistant, or stiffened, *ventricles*.

Remember: Alterations in the resistance, or _____, of   *compliance*
the left ventricular wall produce the first sign of mechanical dys-

function—a rise in _____.   *LVEDP*

Thus gallops are manifestations of a rise in left ventricular _____   *end*

_____ _____.   *diastolic pressure*

94   Gushes of blood enter the ventricles at two times during ventricular diastole: (1) during the *initial* filling phase (early to mid diastole) and (2) at the time of atrial systole (at the *end* of diastole). Gal-

lops thus occur during early and late ventricular _____.   *diastole*

S_3 gallop

95   Ventricular *diastole* begins *after* the closure of the semilunar valves denoted by (S_1/S_2). S_2

The abnormal extra sound created within the ventricles at the *beginning* of ventricular diastole, immediately following the S_2, is known as S_3 *gallop*.

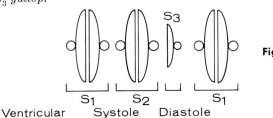

S3

Fig. 7-12

S_1 S_2 S_1

Ventricular   Systole   Diastole

The S$_3$ gallop is heard immediately following _____.   *S$_2$*

Another term used to describe this extra sound is *ventricular* gallop.

S$_4$ gallop

96 Another abnormal sound can occur as the blood enters the ventricles
at the *(beginning/end)* of ventricular diastole. This sound is known   *end*

as an S$_4$ gallop and is associated with _____ systole.   *atrial*

S$_4$ corresponds to _____ systole. Although all gallop sounds are   *atrial*

created in the _____, the S$_4$ gallop, because it is associated   *ventricles*
with atrial systole, is frequently referred to as the atrial gallop.

S$_4$ is heard at the _____ of ventricular diastole, or just *before* _____.   *end*   *S$_1$*

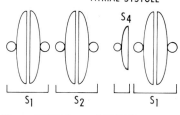

ATRIAL SYSTOLE

S$_4$

Fig. 7-13

S$_1$ S$_2$ S$_1$

VENTRICULAR   SYSTOLE   DIASTOLE

Note: An S$_4$ may occur without the presence of an S$_3$ as it usually
represents an earlier sign of mechanical dysfunction. (See frames
98 to 103.) (Conversely, an S$_3$ may occur without an S$_4$.)

97 The use of the term "gallop" with reference to an S$_3$ or S$_4$ sound
implies that a pathological mechanism is responsible for its production. Either an S$_3$ or S$_4$ sound or both may be present in children or
young adults due to normal ventricular filling. The sounds may become louder during periods of increased ventricular filling such as
with exercise or fever.
With age, however, these sounds usually become dampened and
should not be heard unless ventricular filling is accentuated by the
presence of pathology.

98 *Let us review:* An S$_3$ *gallop* is produced by alterations occurring at
the *(beginning/end)* of ventricular diastole. An S$_4$ *gallop* is pro-   *beginning*
duced by alterations occurring at the *(beginning/end)* of ventricu-   *end*
lar diastole.
The first sign of mechanical dysfunction in acute MI occurs at the
(beginning/end) of ventricular diastole.   *end*
Therefore, the earliest abnormal sound usually heard in acute MI

is an _____ gallop.   *S$_4$*
Any other myocardial pathology that produces alterations in ventricular compliance (thus increasing LVEDP) may also result in
the production of an S$_4$ gallop. Examples include: left ventricular
hypertrophy as occurs with hypertensive disease, the myocardiopa-
thies, and myocardial ischemia occurring during episodes of angina.

99 *Remember:* A *slightly* damaged left ventricle can accommodate
the blood that enters during the initial filling phase, although it

cannot accommodate the added volume that enters with _____   *atrial*
contraction.

162

However, when the presence of heart failure complicates acute MI, the cardiac output falls and the injured left ventricle may not completely eject its contents.

As a result, residual volume remains in the left ventricle at the end

of systole and the beginning of _____.   *diastole*

100 When the above condition is present, the left ventricle cannot fully accommodate the blood that enters even during the initial stages. Thus in the presence of left ventricular failure, an abnormal sound may also be heard at the beginning of diastole.

When an abnormal sound is produced at the *beginning* of diastole,

it is referred to as an _____ gallop. S_3

IN SUMMARY:

101 Gallops may occur as a result of:
  1. *increased blood volume* (larger "gush") producing *(increased/*   *increased*
     decreased) ventricular filling
  2. *stiffened ventricles*, which offer *(more/less)* resistance to filling   *more*
  The patient with left ventricular failure resulting from acute MI

  may have both an increased blood _____ and _____   *volume*   *stiffened*
  ventricles; thus the presence of ventricular gallop sounds in this
  patient *(is/is not)* a common finding.   *is*
  Gallops reflect *(increases/decreases)* in left ventricular diastolic   *increases*
  pressure (LVDP).
  A slight rise in LVEDP *(is/is not)* an expected occurrence in an   *is*
  acute MI. Early increases in LVEDP associated with initial
  changes in compliance are reflected by the presence of an *(S_3/S_4)* S_4
  gallop.
  Thus the presence of an S_4 gallop *(is/is not)* an expected finding   *is*
  in patients with acute MI.
  Further increases in left ventricular diastolic pressure due to left
  ventricular failure *(are/are not)* considered a *complication* of   *are*
  acute MI. These are reflected by the presence of an *(S_3/S_4)* gallop. S_3

102 It is not unusual to find *both* an S_3 and S_4 gallop present in a patient with left ventricular failure resulting from an acute MI. The resulting sound is a *quadruple rhythm.*

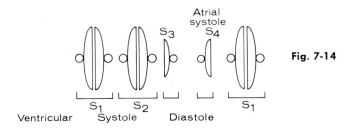

Fig. 7-14

103 *Remember:* A manifestation of CHF is *(fast/slow)* rates. With   *fast*
fast rates, the gallop sounds blend together, producing a summation gallop.

A summation gallop on auscultation sounds like a *galloping horse* —hence its name.

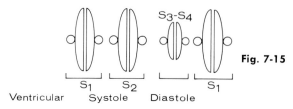

Fig. 7-15

Ventricular   Systole   Diastole

Murmurs

104 The other major abnormal heart sound is a *murmur.* Murmurs occur because of alterations in the movement of blood—its acceleration or deceleration.

Remember: The study of alterations in the movement of blood is

known as _____. Therefore, murmurs *(do/do not)*   *hemodynamics; do*
reflect hemodynamic changes.

105 The movement of blood is significantly altered when there is leakage through insufficient valves or when turbulence occurs across a narrowed outlet as with *stenotic* valves.

Murmurs are labeled according to when they occur—*systolic* or *diastolic.*

Systolic murmurs

106 A *systolic* murmur is heard between the heart sounds S__ and   *1*

S__.   *2*

In *systole,* the A-V valves should be closed and the semilunar

valves should be opened. *Insufficient* _____ valves or *stenotic*   *A-V*

_____ valves, then, may cause systolic murmurs.   *semilunar*

Note: A-V valve (mitral) insufficiency is the most likely cause of murmurs heard in acute MI. This insufficiency is usually due to *papillary muscle dysfunction.* Another possible cause is ventricular *dilation* resulting from congestive heart failure.

Diastolic murmurs

107 If a sudden very loud systolic murmur appears, possible causes are: (1) ruptured interventricular septum or (2) ruptured papillary muscle.

108 A diastolic murmur is heard between the heart sounds S__ and   *2*

S__. In *diastole* the A-V valves should be open and the semilunar   *1*

valves should be closed. Insufficient _____ valves or *ste-*   *semilunar*

notic _____ valves, then, may cause diastolic murmurs.   *A-V*

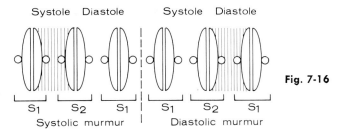

Systole   Diastole   Systole   Diastole

| S_1 | S_2 | S_1 | | S_1 | S_2 | S_1 |

Systolic murmur   Diastolic murmur

Fig. 7-16

NORMAL VARIATIONS OF THE HEART SOUNDS

109 Because of the *dual* component to A-V valve *closure*, the intensity of (S_1/S_2) may be either *loud* or *soft*. (See Unit 1.)

The A-V valves begin closing passively because of increases in ventricular pressure occurring with ventricular filling.

If the A-V valves have had enough time to *start closing* passively before active closure with ventricular systole occurs, the sound of *active*, or *completed*, closure will be *soft*.

If the A-V valves are still wide *open* when ventricular systole begins, the valves will *slam* shut with active closure, producing a

_____ sound.

S_1

loud

LOUD S_1 SOFT S_1

Fig. 7-17

VALVES STILL WIDE OPEN   SOME PASSIVE CLOSURE
WHEN VENTRICULAR   HAS OCCURRED BY THE TIME
CONTRACTION OCCURS   OF VENTRICULAR CONTRACTION

110 Conditions that *shorten* filling time or time for passive closure are:
1. short P-R (0.12 second; i.e., still normal)
2. tachycardia (supraventricular)
3. early beats (for example, early versus late PVC)
The above conditions *(increase/decrease)* passive closure time and therefore produce a *(loud/soft)* S_1.

decrease
loud

111 Conditions that *prolong* filling time or time for passive closure are:

1. long _____
2. *(tachy/brady)*cardia
The above conditions *(increase/decrease)* passive closure time and therefore, produce a *(loud/soft)* S_1.

P-R
brady
increase
soft

112 In CHF there is incomplete emptying of the ventricles during systole. As a result, during diastole there is an increase in ventricular contents.

This increase in contents creates an *(increased/decreased)* pressure against the A-V valves, *enhancing* passive closure. Thus in the setting of CHF a *(loud/soft)* S_1 is heard.

increased

soft

113 *Note: Varying intensity* may indicate rhythms with a varying

P-R rhythm. This is a bedside clue to the diagnosis of *complete heart block* and other forms of A-V *dissociation*. The presence or absence of varying intensity may also aid in the differential diagnosis of *ventricular tachycardia* and *supraventricular tachycardia with aberration*. (See Unit 10.)

114 Let us now discuss the effects of respiration on heart sounds. Inspiration creates a *negative* pressure within the chest. This negative pressure draws blood *(into/out of)* the right side of the heart. Thus there is *increased* filling in the right side of the heart with *(inspiration/expiration)*.

into

inspiration

115 As a result of this increased filling and increased right ventricular contents, right ventricular systole is longer in duration. The *(pulmonary/aortic)* component to S_2 denoting the end of right ventricular systole is therefore delayed and separated from the aortic sound. This creates a splitting of the second heart sound (S_2).

pulmonary

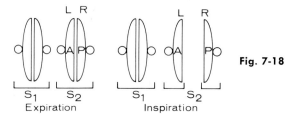

Fig. 7-18

Splitting of S_2 on inspiration, then, *(is/is not)* a normal variation of heart sounds.

is

Note: Splitting is loudest at the second intercostal space.

Conditions that further delay right ventricular systole may augment this normal splitting. Common conditions delaying right ventricular systole include RBBB or a left ventricular pacemaker (caused by delayed right ventricular activation).

116 Anything that delays *left ventricular* systole causes closure of the *aortic valve* to occur with delay. This produces a paradoxical splitting of S_2 on expiration.

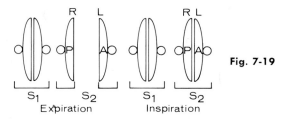

Fig. 7-19

Examples of conditions that delay left ventricular systole are:
1. left ventricular failure
2. LBBB or a right ventricular pacemaker (caused by delayed left ventricular activation)
3. ventricular aneurysm
4. angina pectoris

Paradoxical splitting on expiration *(is/is not)* a normal variation of heart sounds.

is not

117 *Nursing orders:* Auscultation
1. In the patient with an MI, auscultate the heart with each set of vital signs and listen for:

166

- gallop sounds
- murmurs, especially *(systolic/diastolic)*   *systolic*
- changes in the intensity of S_1
- paradoxical splitting of S_2 on *(inspiration/expiration)*   *expiration*

2. Identify the *normal* heart sounds first!
3. When auscultating the heart listen first *at the apex* so that the most significant changes may be heard.
4. When listening for paradoxical splitting of S_2, listen only at the second intercostal space. Do not report *normal* splitting heard on *(inspiration/expiration)*.   *inspiration*
5. When auscultating *gallops:*
   - listen for both S_3 and S_4 during *(systole/diastole)*   *diastole*
   - listen for S_3 together with *(S_1/S_2)*   *S_2*
   - listen for S_4 at the *end* of diastole together with *(S_1/S_2)*   *S_1*
   - listen with light pressure using the bell of the stethoscope; these are low-frequency sounds and are easily obliterated
   - do not expect to hear two distinct sounds; gallops often sound like mere distortions of the normal heart sound
   - left ventricular sounds may be augmented:
     - on expiration
     - with patient in a supine position (increased venous return) on his left side (left ventricle closer to chest wall)
     - with mild strain such as coughing or squeezing the examiner's hand

   (*Remember:* The presence of an S_4 gallop without a concurrent S_3 gallop does *not* indicate CHF.)
6. Report any new murmurs immediately!
   - listen for murmurs, especially between S_1 and S_2 *(systole/*   *systole*
     diastole), as these are the most significant in acute MI
   - if the murmur is loud and the onset is apparently sudden, watch patient closely, checking vital signs until physician has checked patient

   (*Remember:* A sudden loud murmur in the setting of acute MI   *papillary muscle*

   may indicate _____ _____ _____ or   *rupture*

   _____.)   *VSD*

   Be especially concerned in the setting of *anteroseptal* MI with an old inferior MI or vice versa.
   - complete auscultation of a murmur includes noting:
     - whether it is systolic or diastolic
     - if it occurs early, late, or throughout the cycle
     - where it is heard the loudest on the chest
     - where it radiates
     - its quality (e.g., blowing, musical)
     - exactly how loud it is (usually noted on a scale of 1 to 6 with 6 being the loudest; a grade III/VI or IV/VI murmur is a moderately loud one—a beginner should start with these)
7. When hearing *varying intensity* of S_1, look at monitor for an arrhythmia indicating a form of atrioventricular dissociation.

8. If paradoxical splitting is heard, rule out _____,   *aneurysm*

             LBBB; right ven-

   _____ or _____ _____ _____, and   *tricular pacing*

   _____ when considering it as a sign of heart failure.   *angina*
9. Abnormal heart sounds are frequently of very low intensity

and therefore very difficult to hear. When first starting to listen, ask another nurse or physician to verify your findings. Ability to hear these changes accurately develops only with practice.

THE SHOCK SYNDROME

118 The shock syndrome may be defined as a state in which there is a *significant* fall in cardiac output resulting in a decreased supply of oxygenated blood to the tissues and *tissue symptoms.*

119 In the presence of heart failure resulting from an acute MI there *(is/is not)* a fall in cardiac output.
        is
Therefore, CHF due to an acute MI has the *potential,* if *the patient's condition* deteriorates, to lead to a *symptomatic* fall in cardiac output, or *shock.*
There are, however, other mechanisms that may lead to the shock state in the presence of an acute MI. These should also be recognized and taken into consideration.

120 Shock is a clinical syndrome that occurs as a result of acute circulatory failure. The common denominator to all forms of shock is a *critical reduction* in the supply of oxygenated blood to the tissues.
Remember: The demands of the tissues for oxygen are met by an adequate oxygen supply and an adequate blood supply.

Tissue demands (oxygen consumption) = _____ _____   *blood supply*

(cardiac output) × _____ _____ (oxygen content).   *oxygen supply*

121 Maintenance of an adequate blood supply is dependent upon the integrity of the cardiovascular system. (See Fig. 7-1.)
The integrity of the cardiovascular system is affected by any of *four* variables:
1. heart rate and rhythm

2. blood _____   *volume*
3. vascular resistance, or *tone*

4. cardiac muscle _____   *contractility*

122 Evaluation of the *blood pressure* is a useful clinical tool for the initial assessment of cardiovascular function.
Blood pressure = cardiac output × peripheral vascular resistance.
A fall in blood pressure usually accompanies the shock state.

123 Significant alterations of any of the above four variables may

cause a marked decrease in the supply of oxygenated _____ to   *blood*

the _____. This is reflected by a significant fall in _____   *tissues; blood*
pressure, changes in cellular metabolism, and a group of characteristic

symptoms. This clinical *syndrome* is known as _____.   *shock*

124 A shock-like state may occur as a result of a tachyarrhythmia or

a _____arrhythmia.   *brady-*
Remember: CO = stroke volume × _____ _____.   *heart rate*
In the setting of coronary care, all possible causes of a shock state must be considered.

125 *Hypovolemic* shock may result from a severe reduction in the

_____ _____.   *blood volume*
Excessive diuresis and a resultant *(increased/decreased)* blood vol-   *decreased*
ume may cause shock.

126 *Vasogenic* shock may result from a decrease in vascular resistance,

or _____. Drugs that produce vasodilation, such as morphine   *tone*

or certain sympathetic blockers, may contribute to _____   *vasogenic*
shock. (See Unit 8.) The problem of sepsis and endotoxic shock
should also be considered when assessing *(increased/decreased)*   *decreased*
vascular tone.

127 *Cardiogenic* shock results from *severe* impairment of cardiac muscle contractility. In the setting of *cardiogenic* shock caused by
coronary artery disease 40% or more of the myocardium is ne-
crotic or injured and as such *(does/does not)* contribute to con-   *does not*
tractility. By definition, therefore, cardiogenic shock implies the
presence of extensive muscle damage. The prognosis is extremely
(poor/good) and the mortality rate is high.   *poor*

128 With early, aggressive clinical intervention, the area of myocardial infarction may be contained. Without appropriate clinical
management, however, areas of *critically ischemic* tissue may subsequently become necrotic, thus extending the area of infarction.
At this point signs of heart failure may begin to evolve into

cardiogenic _____.   *shock*

129 The development of shock in a cardiac patient must be assessed

from all parameters: rhythm, blood _____, vascular _____,   *volume*   *tone*

and cardiac muscle _____. Initial therapy should be di-   *contractility*
rected toward correcting disturbances in rhythm, volume, and

vascular _____. If these measures are ineffective and no *recog-*   *tone*
nizable or *treatable* cause of the shock state can be identified, the

diagnosis of _____ shock is made.   *cardiogenic*

130 Shock is a clinical syndrome that occurs as a result of acute

_____ failure. The common denominator in all forms of   *circulatory*

shock is a critical reduction in supply of _____ _____   *oxygenated blood*
to the tissues. This results in *(adequate/inadequate)* tissue per-   *inadequate*
fusion.

131 The clinical picture of a patient in shock is a reflection of three
major occurrences:
1. the inadequate blood supply to the body's tissues
2. the compensatory mechanisms of the body resulting in changes
   in the microcirculation
3. the response at the cellular level

132 When the blood supply to the tissues is inadequate, a series of
compensatory mechanisms is initiated in order to maintain an ade-

quate blood supply to the _____, _____ and _____.   *heart; brain; kidney*
The most important compensatory mechanisms are:

1. *(increased/decreased)* heart rate

   Remember: One reflection of the blood supply to the tissues is

   the blood _____.

   BP = _____ _____ × peripheral resistance; CO =

   stroke volume × _____ _____.

2. constriction of the blood vessels to the _____, abdominal vis-

   cera, voluntary muscles, and finally even the _____.

   These compensatory mechanisms occur as a result of *sympathetic*
   stimulation.

increased

pressure

cardiac output

heart rate
skin

kidneys

133 The symptoms of acute circulatory failure include:

heart—*(increased/decreased)* heart _____
skin—cool and moist (clammy)
kidneys—decreased urine output to *oliguria* or *anuria*
brain—lethargy, dizziness, confusion, agitation

increased   rate

134 The decreased supply of oxygenated blood to the tissues triggers

_____ mechanisms that cause vasoconstriction in

the _____ and _____.
The skin assumes a dusky, cool, moist appearance.
The fall in cardiac output and the vasoconstriction of the vessels
to the kidneys cause *(increased/decreased)* renal perfusion, which

results in oliguria or _____.

compensatory

kidneys   skin

decreased

anuria

135 In spite of the compensatory mechanisms, there is a(n) *(in-
creased/decreased)* supply of oxygenated blood to the brain resulting in *(increased/decreased)* cerebral perfusion. Decreased perfusion to the brain is manifested by *sensorium changes* such as dizziness, confusion, agitation, lethargy.
These changes may further progress to a state of *coma*.

decreased
decreased

136 The precise clinical picture of the patient in shock may vary. It is
dependent upon the *cause* of the disorder and the *stage* of the
shock.

137 Let us now consider the changes that occur in *microcirculation*—
at the capillary level— and the response of the *cells*.
In the presence of normal circulation, the capillary bed is perfused.
The arterial and venous links to the capillary bed are open.

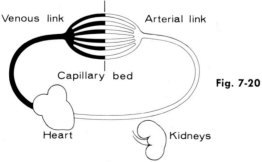

Fig. 7-20

138 With a decrease in systemic blood pressure, the compensatory
mechanisms respond by releasing sympathetic chemicals—*epi-*

nephrine and *norepinephrine*. These hormones attempt to restrict blood flow to the tissues by *(vasoconstriction/vasodilation)*. Blood is shunted from the kidneys, mesentery, and extremities to the

vasoconstriction

more critical areas of the _____ and _____.
The arterial and venous links to the capillary bed are *(constricted/dilated)*. This constriction prevents adequate circulation through the capillary bed. This decrease in circulation implies a decrease in oxygen supply as well.

brain   heart
constricted

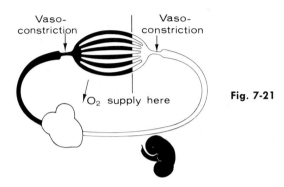

Fig. 7-21

139 The inadequate cellular perfusion causes cell *anoxia* and changes in cellular *metabolism*. During cellular anoxia, the cells are forced to metabolize glucose *(with/without)* oxygen. This abnormal metabolic process is described as *anaerobic metabolism*. As a result,

without

_____ _____ accumulates within the cell.

lactic acid

140 Metabolic acidosis develops, which results in a(n) *(increase/decrease)* in serum pH levels. The arterial ends of the capillary bed are not accustomed to an *(acidic/alkaline)* environment and as a result vasodilation occurs. The venous link from the capillary bed, however, remains *(dilated/constricted)*. Therefore, blood flows into the capillary bed, but cannot return to the heart. Stasis

decrease
acidic

constricted

and pooling of large volumes of _____ occur in the capillary bed. At this point, *cellular*, *tissue*, and *organ* death is imminent.

blood

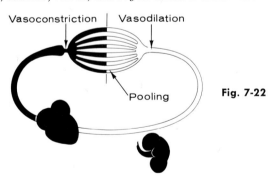

Fig. 7-22

141 Therapy of shock is based upon three principles: (1) treatment of the underlying cause, (2) evaluation of the vascular response, (3) assisting tissue metabolism.
Remember: The common denominator of all forms of shock is a

critical reduction in the supply of _____ _____ to

oxygenated blood

the tissues, resulting in inadequate tissue _____. The

perfusion

171

goal of shock therapy, then, is to restore adequate tissue

_____. *perfusion*

Therapy of the shock state is directed toward correcting possible causes:

1. correcting any disturbances in _____ *rhythm*

2. correcting disturbances in _____ *volume*

3. increasing vascular _____ *tone*

4. improving myocardial _____ *contractility*

142 Further management of a shock state is dependent upon the stage of the shock and the ability of the blood vessels to respond. Generally, shock therapy may include:
1. administering drugs to correct disturbances in rhythm
2. administering appropriate amounts and types of intravenous fluids
3. administering drugs that increase vascular tone *and/or* promote microcirculation
4. administering drugs that improve myocardial contractility
5. administering drugs that assist tissue metabolism
6. monitoring of various *physiologic parameters:* central venous pressure, urine output, cardiac rhythm, arterial blood gases, PA and wedge pressure, and cardiac output

CARDIOGENIC SHOCK

143 *Let us review:* The mechanism of the shock state is determined to

be cardiogenic in origin only after any problem in _____, *rhythm*

_____, or _____ _____ has been corrected. *volume; vascular tone*

Therapy of shock is based upon three principles: (1) treatment of *underlying cause;*
 vascular
the _____ _____, (2) evaluation of the _____

response, and (3) assisting _____ metabolism. *tissue*

144 Cardiogenic shock results from severe impairment of cardiac muscle contractility. (See frames 127 and 128.)
Although cardiogenic shock represents a decreased contractile state, increasing myocardial contractility is not the immediate goal of therapy.
The use of inotropic agents such as digitalis or isoproterenol (Isuprel) may be potentially hazardous because the increase in contractility is accompanied by a(n) *(increased/decreased)* oxygen *increased*
consumption. The net result may be an extension of the area of infarction.

145 In cardiogenic shock resulting from coronary artery disease, the impairment of contractile function results from dicrepancies in myocardial oxygen supply and demand. The initial goal in the treatment of coronary cardiogenic shock is limiting or decreasing this discrepancy, thus improving myocardial oxygenation.
Therapy should be directed toward maintaining the demands for myocardial oxygen consumption at a minimum and improving the

coronary blood _____. *supply*

146 *Initial* therapy is directed toward limiting the myocardial *demands.*

Let us review: The determinants of myocardial oxygen *demands* (MVO$_2$) are:
1. the heart's *rate*
2. the heart's *preload,* or volume of filling
3. the heart's *afterload,* or the peripheral vascular resistance
4. the myocardial *contractility*

Thus measures that limit or decrease myocardial demands include:
1. control of heart rhythm and _____   *rate*
2. limiting ventricular filling to decrease the heart's _____;   *preload*
   (this is best accomplished while concurrently monitoring ventricular filling pressure with a Swan-Ganz catheter)
3. lowering the peripheral vascular resistance, as with vasodilators, to decrease the heart's _____   *afterload*
4. limiting or lowering *tissue* demands in an attempt to decrease demands for myocardial *contractility*
   Remember: Tissue oxygen consumption = blood supply (cardiac output) × oxygen supply.

147 Myocardial oxygen consumption *demands* may be lowered by the use of *vasodilator therapy.*
Coronary blood supply may be improved by:
1. surgical revascularization
2. the use of vasoconstricting agents
All three parameters of coronary cardiogenic shock—*cardiac output,* myocardial demands, and coronary blood *supply*—may be improved by the *circulatory assist* measures.

148 *Remember:* The coronary arteries receive their blood supply during *(systole/diastole).*   *diastole*
Thus increasing coronary blood supply can be accomplished by *augmenting* arterial diastolic pressure.
Drugs and circulatory assist measures that increase coronary blood flow by increasing diastolic pressure are frequently referred
to as modes of diastolic _____.   *augmentation*

149 Pharmacological *vasoconstrictors* such as norepinephrine (Levophed) increase arterial and venous peripheral resistance. Therefore, they augment both arterial and venous diastolic pressure.
Coronary blood flow is *(increased/decreased).* Norepinephrine also   *increased*
supports the body's compensatory response by extending sites of
(vasodilation/vasoconstriction).   *vasoconstriction*

150 Increased arterial peripheral vascular resistance also results in an undesirable increase in the heart's *(preload/afterload).*   *afterload*
The increased *venous* resistance and enhanced venous return results in an increase in the heart's filling, or *(preload/afterload).*   *preload*
Thus myocardial oxygen consumption may be *(increased/*   *increased*
decreased), and extension of the area of infarction may result.

151 For this reason a popular approach in the current management of coronary cardiogenic shock is the use of *vasodilating* agents.
Both arterial and venous resistance are lowered by vasodilators such as Nitroprusside. Nitroprusside *(increases/decreases)* both   *decreases*
the preload and afterload and *(increases/decreases)* myocardial   *decreases*
oxygen consumption.
Since arterial diastolic pressure is reduced, coronary blood flow

may be *(increased/decreased)*. However, this effect is usually off-set by the decreased myocardial demands.

decreased

152 Lowering of the afterload by arterial vasodilation reduces the impedence to left ventricular ejection, facilitating ventricular systole. Thus the cardiac output is *(improved/reduced)*.

improved

153 Although the coronary blood supply is not increased, vasodilator therapy appears to have the unique advantage of improving cardiac output while at the same time *lowering* myocardial demands. However, the *ideal* mode of therapy should act to improve all *three* parameters of coronary cardiogenic shock:
1. improve cardiac output
2. lower myocardial demands
3. increase coronary blood flow
Circulatory assist measures provide this beneficial three-fold effect.

Circulatory assist measures

154 The modes of circulatory assist act to increase coronary blood flow by augmenting diastole.
They, therefore, act by the principle of _____ _____.

diastolic augmentation

Systolic pressure, however, is concurrently *reduced* by producing a decrease in the arterial vascular resistance, or the heart's *(preload/afterload)*. Systolic emptying is thus facilitated and the cardiac output is *(increased/decreased)*.

afterload
increased

155 This lowering of systolic and increasing of diastolic pressure represents a *counterpulsation* as compared with the heart's natural pulsation.
Therapeutic methods resulting in such an effect are also known as

modes of _____.

counterpulsation

156 The most popular mode of counterpulsation in current use is the *intra-aortic balloon pump.*
The intra-aortic balloon catheter is inserted through the femoral artery into the aorta. Inflation and deflation of the balloon are usually synchronized to the R wave of the ECG. However, they may also be adjusted to the arterial pulse wave.
Inflation of the balloon during diastole results in *(augmentation/reduction)* of coronary blood flow.

augmentation

Deflation of the intra-aortic balloon just prior to systole exerts an almost sucking effect allowing for more complete and easier evacuation of the left ventricle during systole.

157 Evaluation of the effectiveness of the balloon pump is made by observation of characteristic changes in the pressure pulse pattern.
(See The pressure pulse patterns, p. 154.)

THE INTRA-AORTIC BALLOON PUMP

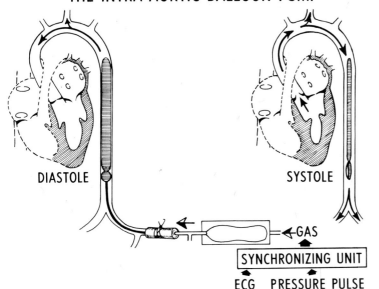

DIASTOLE   SYSTOLE

←GAS

SYNCHRONIZING UNIT

ECG   PRESSURE PULSE

Fig. 7-23

TRACE:

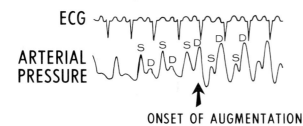

ECG

ARTERIAL
PRESSURE

ONSET OF AUGMENTATION

Note: The balloon appears to be inflating during systole if compared with the timing of the QRS complex. However, remember
that *mechanical* systole begins slightly *after* the onset of electrical
systole—at about the peak of the QRS complex.

158 Intra-aortic counterpulsation produces hemodynamic changes that
favorably alter the relationship between oxygen supply and demand in the severely impaired myocardium.
Use of the intra-aortic balloon may reverse the shock state or serve
to stabilize the patient in preparation for cardiac catheterization
and possible coronary artery surgery.

159 *Nursing orders:* Shock and circulatory assist
1. Evaluate *underlying cause*
— place patient in flat position
— treat *arrhythmias* or other abnormalities evident on ECG
— check for *hypovolemia*
     — elevate legs to increase venous return; then:
     — check blood pressure
     — check CVP, pulmonary artery pressures, and wedge pres-
       sure
— monitor vital signs closely
— remove any rotating tourniquets

— have resuscitation equipment at the bedside
— rule out any vasoactive mechanism such as morphine, Demerol, nitroglycerine, or sepsis
  — elevate legs to increase venous return
  — have narcotic antagonists available
— if possible, monitor cardiac output accurately by indicator-dilution technique (otherwise, evaluate *changes* in cardiac output by comparison of arterial and venous blood gases)
— *if mechanism is determined to be cardiogenic and is associated with coronary artery disease*—institute measure to limit discrepancy between myocardial oxygen supply and demand
— nursing action limiting myocardial oxygen consumption:
  — *rate:* watch for and correct any significant arrhythmias quickly
  — *preload:* monitor fluid intake and output carefully; administer diuretics as ordered; check wedge pressure for effectiveness
  — *afterload:* correct any hypertensive state; relieve stress factors such as pain or anxiety
  — *contractility:* correct any acid/base or electrolyte abnormalities quickly; limit peripheral demands by providing and investigating and/or managing any other systemic diseases such as diabetes, chronic lung disease, sepsis; if inotropic agents are ordered, monitor vital signs and other hemodynamic parameters carefully for patient deterioration
— nursing action increasing oxygen supply:
  — administer supplementary oxygen; be sure to document effectiveness on blood gases
2. Evaluate *vascular response:*
   — monitor vasoactive drugs carefully (Levophed, Aramine, Dopamine, Nitroprusside; see Unit 8)
   — determine end point of therapy with physician
3. Evaluate and assist *tissue metabolism*
   — monitor blood gases for metabolic acidosis
   — watch for Kussmaul-type respirations as sign of respiratory compensatory efforts
   — evaluate patient symptoms of tissue perfusion; watch for deterioration such as deepening of sensorium changes
   — administer and monitor effects of drugs that may aid in stabilizing tissue metabolism, such as steroids or osmotic diuretics
4. When *circulatory assist* measures are instituted:
   — monitor effectiveness of diastolic augmentation by evaluating arterial pressure pulse pattern
   — monitor inflation and deflation of slave balloon with intra-aortic balloon pump
     — watch dressing at graft site for bleeding
   — begin to titrate vasoactive agents accordingly
   — compare pressure pattern with ECG pattern to determine if augmentation is occurring at appropriate time
   — watch for loss of augmentation with arrhythmias
   — administer anticoagulant agents as ordered to prevent development of clots at balloon site

Suggested readings

Ayres, S., and Mueller, H.: The overall approach to the patient with hypertension, Heart Lung, May-June 1974.

Beland, I. L.: Clinical nursing; pathophysiology and psychosocial approaches, New York, 1967, The Macmillan Co.

Bordicks, K. J.: Patterns of shock—implications for nursing care, New York, 1966, The Macmillan Co.

Braumwald, E., and Maroko, P. K.: The reduction of infarct size—an idea whose time (for testing) has come, Circulation 50:206, Aug. 1974.

Bristow, J. D., and Metcalfe, J.: Physical signs in congestive heart failure, Prog. Cardiov. Dis. 10:236, 1967.

Broder, M. I., and Cohn, J. N.: Evaluation of abnormalities in left ventricular function after acute myocardial infarction, Circulation 46:731, Oct. 1972.

Broughton, J. O.: Chest physical diagnosis for nurses and respiratory therapists, Heart Lung 1(2):201, Mar.-Apr. 1972.

Chatterjee, K., and others: Hemodynamic and metabolic responses to vasodilator therapy in acute myocardial infarction, Circulation 48:1183, Dec. 1973.

Corday, E., and others: Physiologic principles in the application of circulatory assist for the failing heart, Am. J. Cardiol. 26:595, Dec. 1970.

Corday, E., and others: Treatment of cardiogenic shock with mechanical circulatory assist—fact or fiction Am. J. Cardiol. 30:575, Oct. 1972.

Craige, E.: Gallop rhythm, Prog. Cardiov. Dis. 10:247, 1967.

Dunkman, B. W., and others: Clinical and hemodynamic results of intra-aortic balloon pumping and surgery for cardiogenic shock, Circulation 46:465, Sept. 1972.

Durie, M. E.: Use of an intra-aortic balloon pump following postoperative pump failure and cardiac arrest: Case presentation and discussion, Heart Lung 3(6):971, Nov.-Dec. 1974.

Edwards, J. C.: The value and limitations of necropsy studies in coronary artery disease, Prog. Cardiov. Dis. 13:309, 1971.

Ellis, R. J., and others: Computerized monitoring of cardiac output by thermal dilution, J.A.M.A. 220:4, April 24, 1972.

Forrester, J. S., Diamond, G. A., and Swan, H. J. C.: Bedside diagnosis of latent cardiac complications in acutely ill patients, J.A.M.A 222(1):59, October 2, 1972.

Forrester, J. S., and Swan, H. J. C.: Optimal level of filling pressure in the left side of the heart in acute myocardial infarction, New Engl. J. Med. 280:1263-1266, 1973.

Forsberg, S. A.: Relations between pressure in pulmonary artery, left atrium, and left ventricle with special reference to events at end diastole, Br. Heart J. 33:494-499, 1971.

Foster, S. B.: Pump failure, Am. J. Nurs. Oct. 1974.

Frazee, S., and Nail, L.: New challenge in cardiac nursing: The intra-aortic balloon, Heart Lung 2(4):526, July-Aug. 1973.

Friedberg, C. K.: Diseases of the heart, Philadelphia, 1966, W. B. Saunders Co.

Gamong, W. F.: Review of medical physiology, Los Altos, Calif., 1969, Lange Medical Publications.

Grace, W. J., and Keyoun, V.: The coronary care unit, New York, 1970, Appleton-Century-Crofts.

Guyton, A. C.: Textbook of medical physiology, Philadelphia, 1971, W. B. Saunders Co.

Hurst, W. J., and Logue, R. B.: editors: The heart arteries and veins, New York, 1970, McGraw-Hill Book Co.

Karliner, J. S., and Ross, J.: Left ventricular performance after acute myocardial infarction, Prog. Cardiov. Dis. 13:374-387, 1971.

Kroetz, F. W., Leon, D. F., and Leonard, J. J.: The diagnosis of acute circulatory failure; shock and syncope, Prog. Cardiov. Dis. 10:262, 1967.

Leonard, J. J., and Kroetz, F. W.: Examination of the heart. Part IV, Auscultation, New York, 1966, The American Heart Association.

Lillehei, R. C., and others: Nature of irreversible shock; experimental and clinical observations, Ann. Surg. 160:682, 1964.

Lillehei, R. C., and others: The modern treatment of shock based on physiologic principles, Clin. Pharm. Ther. 5:63, 1964.

Lillehei, C. W., and Carlsen, R. O.: Surgical treatment of ventricular failure due to coronary artery insufficiency, Heart Lung 1(1):90, Jan.-Feb. 1972.

Luisada, A. A.: The sounds of the normal heart, St. Louis, 1972, Warren H. Green, Inc.

Luisada, A. A.: Changing views on the mechanism of the first and second heart sounds, Am. Heart J. 88(4):503, Oct. 1974.

Netter, F. H.: Heart—The Ciba Collection of Medical Illustrations, Summit, N. J., 1969, Ciba Publications.

Nielsen, M. A.: Intra-arterial monitoring of blood pressure, Am. J. Nurs. Jan. 1974.

Perloff, J. K., Talano, J. V., and Roman, J. A.: Non-invasive techniques in acute myocardial infarction, Prog. Cardiov. Dis. 13:437, 1971.

Prior, J. A., and Silberstein, J. S.: Physical diagnosis—the history and examination of the patient, St. Louis, 1973, The C. V. Mosby Co.

Rodbard, S.: The clinical utility of the arterial pulses and sounds, Heart Lung 1(6):776, Nov.-Dec. 1972.

Rotman, M., and Gilbert, M. R.: Pulmonary artery diastolic pressure in acute myocardial infarction, Am. J. Cardiol. 33:3, Mar. 1974.

Rushmer, R. T.: Cardiovascular dynamics, Philadelphia, 1970, W. B. Saunders Co.

Russell, R. O., Jr., and others: Left ventricular hemodynamics in anterior and inferior myocardial infarction, Am. J. Cardiol. 32:1, July 1973.

Sampson, J. J., and Hutchinson, J. C.: Heart failure in myocardial infarction, Prog. Cardiov. Dis. 10:1, 1967.

Scheidt, S., and others: Intra-aortic balloon counter-pulsation in cardiogenic shock, New Engl. J. Med. 228:19, May 1973.

Segal, B. L., editor: The theory and practice of auscultation, Philadelphia, 1964, F. A. Davis.

Shock: recognition and management, Philadelphia, 1968, Smith, Kline & French Laboratories.

Soderman, W. A.: Pathologic physiology, ed. 4, Philadelphia, 1968, W. B. Saunders Co.

Sonnenblick, E. H.: Oxygen consumption of the heart: Physiologic principles and clinical implications, Mod. Con. Cardiovas. Dis. 40:3, Mar. 1971.

Swan, H. J. C., Ganz, W., Forrester, J., and others: Catheterization of the heart in man with the use of a flow-directed balloon-tipped catheter, New Engl. J. Med. 283:447, 1970.

Traver, G.: Assessment of the thorax and lungs, Am. J. Nurs. Mar. 1973, pp. 466-471.

The shock syndrome: pathogenesis and management, Kalamazoo, Mich., 1967, The Upjohn Co.

Wartak, J.: Phonocardiology: Integrated study of heart sounds and murmurs, New York, 1972, Harper and Row Publishers.

Welch, W. J.: Medical aspects of congestive heart failure, Cardiov. Nurs. 3:3, 1967.

Pharmacological intervention in acute myocardial infarction

1 In the setting of acute myocardial infarction, there are four major problems that may complicate the clinical course:
1. chest pain
2. arrhythmias
3. heart failure
4. shock

The use of pharmacological agents in the management of these problems is discussed in this unit.

DRUG THERAPY IN THE MANAGEMENT OF CHEST PAIN

2 The group of drugs most commonly used in the management of the chest pain of acute MI are the narcotic analgesics. Therapy is directed toward relieving the discomfort rapidly and effectively with as few side effects as possible. The two narcotics probably used most commonly in the setting of coronary care are morphine sulfate (morphine) and meperidine hydrochloride (Demerol).

Morphine sulfate

3 Morphine is a central nervous system (CNS) depressant that exerts a *narcotic* effect. A drug that exerts a narcotic effect may produce sleep as well as analgesia. Another manifestation of the narcotic effect may be changes in sensorium. Because of its ability to rapidly and effectively relieve pain when administered intravenously, morphine is commonly used in the management of chest pain associated with acute MI.

4 Another manifestation of the CNS effect of morphine may be vasodilation due to depression of sympathetic pathways.
Thus morphine administration may result in *(hypotension/hypertension)*.

hypotension

5 Morphine has been shown not only to decrease arteriolar constriction but also to produce venodilation.
Venodilation results in peripheral pooling and thus reduces *(preload/afterload)*.
This effect on preload is desirable in the relief of pulmonary congestion in pulmonary edema.

preload

6 Another effect of morphine that is beneficial in the management of pulmonary edema is its ability to decrease the respiratory rate and decrease anxiety.

7 Morphine has also been shown to slow the heart rate in some settings by creating autonomic imbalance. Therefore, morphine should be administered with caution in patients with bradyarrhythmias or enhanced vagal tone such as occurs in *(AWMI/IWMI)*.

IWMI

179

8 Morphine decreases the sensitivity of the respiratory center to arterial CO_2 levels, thereby *(depressing/stimulating)* respirations. *depressing*
The administration of morphine in patients with known limited respiratory reserves must, therefore, be approached with caution.

Demerol (meperidine hydrochloride)

9 Demerol, another narcotic analgesic, is structurally different from morphine but has a similar mechanism of action.
Because of its ability to rapidly and effectively relieve pain when administered intravenously, it is also commonly used in the management of chest pain associated with acute MI.

10 Demerol depresses respirations by decreasing the tidal volume rather than by depressing the respiratory rate.

11 Hypotension may occur after the intravenous administration with a compensatory increase in the heart rate.

12 *Nursing orders:* The patient receiving morphine or Demerol
   1. Watch for hypotension following intravenous administration.
      — elevate legs as indicated
   2. Observe for respiratory depression following administration.
      — administer with caution in patients with known limited respiratory reserve, i.e., emphysema, asthma, bronchitis, pneumonia
   3. Administer morphine with caution in the patient with increased vagal tone; have atropine available.
      — IWMI
      — bradyarrhythmia
   4. The following side effects may occur with the administration of morphine or Demerol:
      — dizziness
      — sweating
      — nausea and vomiting
      — weakness
      — syncope
      — palpitations
      — euphoria or dysphoria

Nitroglycerin

13 Another group of pharmacological agents that may be used to manage chest pain associated with coronary artery disease are the peripheral vasodilators. The most common vasodilator in use is nitroglycerin. Other drugs of the nitrate family are also used for similar effects.

14 *Let us review:* Myocardial infarction is death, or _____, of *necrosis* cardiac muscle resulting from a diminished supply of oxygenated blood.
Another syndrome that results from a *less severe* inadequacy of

blood supply to the myocardium is known as _____ _____. *angina pectoris*
The pain of *angina pectoris* is usually rapidly relieved by administration of *nitroglycerin.*

15 In the presence of coronary artery disease there is a discrepancy between myocardial oxygen supply and demand.
Nitroglycerin enhances myocardial blood supply and lowers myocar-

dial oxygen demands, although the predominant effect is to *reduce demands*.

16 Nitroglycerin may enhance coronary blood flow by relaxing the smooth muscle of the coronary vessels.
It reduces demands by producing arterial and venous dilation. By lowering arterial resistance, the *(afterload/preload)* is reduced. By lowering venous resistance, the *(afterload/preload)* is reduced.

afterload
preload

17 *Nursing orders:* The patient receiving nitroglycerin
1. Watch for episodes of symptomatic hypotension following administration.
   — elevate legs
   — put head of bed down
2. Caution patient to report chest pain unrelieved by three successive tablets taken at about 5 minute intervals.
   Caution patient that nitroglycerin tablets may deteriorate and may lose effectiveness in as short a time as three months.
   — potent tablets characteristically produce a transient headache because of meningeal vasodilation and/or burning sensation under the tongue
   — instruct patient to store nitroglycerin in opaque bottle in refrigerator to protect from light; a few may be carried with the patient for PRN use

DRUG THERAPY IN THE MANAGEMENT OF ARRHYTHMIAS

18 Generally, arrhythmias may be considered as resulting from disturbances in _____ and _____.
The three major types of arrhythmias we will consider are:
1. ventricular arrhythmias
2. fast supraventricular arrhythmias
3. bradyarrhythmias

automaticity; conduction

Ventricular arrhythmias

19 Ventricular arrhythmias are a manifestation of abnormal electrical activity in the _____. Abnormal electrical activity in the ventricles may result in premature ventricular contractions,

ventricles

ventricular tachycardia, or _____ _____.
Remember: Initial therapy in the management of ventricular arrhythmias is directed toward depressing ectopic impulse formation

ventricular fibrillation

in the _____.

ventricles

Antiarrhythmic drugs

20 The drugs used to manage ventricular arrhythmias are known as the *antiarrhythmic drugs.*
The following drugs will be considered in the classification:
1. lidocaine (Xylocaine)
2. quinidine sulfate (Quinidine)
3. procaine amide (Pronestyl)
4. diphenylhydantoin (Dilantin)
5. propranolol (Inderal)
Note: Although the exact mechanism of action of each drug may differ, as a group these drugs act to depress ectopic impulse formation in the ventricles. Some of these drugs also depress ectopic impulse formation in the atria.

21 The drug used most commonly in the management of acute ventricular arrhythmias is *lidocaine* (Xylocaine). Lidocaine is ideal for use in the setting of acute MI because of two characteristics: (1) rapid onset of action, and (2) relative lack of toxic effects on the heart.
Note: Lidocaine does not appear to be useful in the suppression of supraventricular arrhythmias.

22 The effect of lidocaine is to depress ectopic impulse formation in the *ventricles*. In addition to this effect, lidocaine also has an effect on A-V conduction. Although the exact effect is unknown, lidocaine appears to accelerate A-V conduction in the early stages of therapy.
Note: Because lidocaine is a cardiac *(depressant/stimulant)*, it *(would/would not)* be indicated for ventricular arrhythmias that arise in the presence of slow rates.

    depressant
    would not

The route of administration of lidocaine in the acute setting is intravenous. This drug may be given in a single bolus form or via a continuous infusion drip.

23 Common side effects associated with the use of lidocaine are *hypotension* and *sensorium changes*. Alterations in sensorium may range from drowsiness, restlessness, and apprehension to psychosis and convulsions.
In the presence of lidocaine toxicity, *discontinue all* lidocaine.

24 *Let us review:* Lidocaine acts by depressing ectopic impulse formation in the _____.

    ventricles

Lidocaine *(is/is not)* indicated in the therapy of premature ventricular contractions.

    is

Lidocaine *(is/is not)* indicated in the therapy of ventricular tachycardia.

    is

Lidocaine *(may/may not)* be used to prevent the recurrence of ventricular fibrillation.

    may

Common side effects associated with lidocaine are: (1) *(hypotension/hypertension)*, and (2) changes in _____.

    hypotension
    sensorium

25 *Nursing orders:* The patient receiving lidocaine
1. Analyze the need for the drug within the clinical context of the arrhythmia.
  — Is the underlying rhythm *fast or slow?*
  — Is the arrhythmia life threatening?
  — Is the arrhythmia a precursor to a lethal arrhythmia?
Remember: Lidocaine may also be used to prevent the recurrence of _____ _____.

    ventricular fibrillation

2. Evaluate the possible causes of the ventricular arrhythmia (See Unit 5, frame 115.)
3. Monitor cardiac status, blood pressure, and sensorium during intravenous infusion of lidocaine.
  — Evaluate the response of the rhythm to the drug—has the lidocaine therapy suppressed the arrhythmia?
  — Observe the patient for signs of lidocaine toxicity: *(hypotension/hypertension)* and changes in _____.

    hypotension
    sensorium

26 Quinidine and Pronestyl (procaine amide) are grouped together in

this discussion because they have certain *common* actions. Pharmacologically, however, these two drugs are different.

Quinidine sulfate and procaine amide act by depressing ectopic impulse formation in both the atria and the ventricles. Therefore, these drugs may be used in the *acute* or *chronic* management of

both _____ and _____ arrhythmias.   *atrial   ventricular*

27   Quinidine and Pronestyl cause prolongation of the refractory period. Specifically, quinidine produces a U wave and T-U fusion. The ECG manifestation of the quinidine "effect" mimics the ECG pattern of *(hypokalemia/hyperkalemia)*.   *hypokalemia*

These ECG changes indicate the *effect* of quinidine and Pronestyl on the ECG and *(are/are not)* an indication for discontinuing therapy.   *are not*

Another characteristic of quinidine is its ability to accelerate A-V conduction with *initial* administration, especially in the presence of atrial fibrillation. Quinidine is thus said to have a *vagolytic* effect in early stages of therapy.

28   Quinidine and Pronestyl toxicity will be manifested on the ECG as *widening* of the QRS complex. This type of ECG change indicates quinidine or Pronestyl toxicity and *(is/is not)* an indication for discontinuing therapy.   *is*

Note: Some other conditions that produce widening of the QRS are hyperkalemia, complete left bundle branch block, and peri-infarction block. Quinidine and Pronestyl should be administered with *caution* in the presence of left bundle branch block and peri-infarction block.

Remember: Potassium is a cardiac *(depressant/stimulant)*. Therefore, quinidine and Pronestyl would be *contraindicated* in the presence of hyperkalemia. The antidote for quinidine and Pronestyl toxicity is *sodium bicarbonate*. Both the sodium and the alkalotic effect of the bicarbonate exert a stimulating effect on electrical conduction, which reverses the toxic ECG effects of these drugs.   *depressant*

A characteristic of Pronestyl is that it is a *peripheral vasodilator*. Therefore, a side effect associated with the intravenous administration of Pronestyl is _____.   *hypotension*

Quinidine and Pronestyl may also cause gastrointestinal symptoms such as nausea and vomiting. Quinidine frequently causes diarrhea.

29   *Let us review:* The "effect" of quinidine and Pronestyl on the ECG is to *(prolong/shorten)* the refractory period and repolarization.   *prolong*

Specifically, quinidine produces a(n) _____ wave and _____ fusion.   *U   T-U*

Quinidine and Pronestyl may be used in the management of acute or chronic _____ and _____ arrhythmias.   *atrial   ventricular*

Quinidine and Pronestyl toxicity will be manifested on the ECG as *(widening/narrowing)* of the QRS complex.   *widening*

Quinidine and Pronestyl should be administered with caution in the presence of _____ and _____ _____.   *LBBB; peri-infarction block*

Quinidine and Pronestyl are contraindicated in the presence of *(hypo-/hyper-)*kalemia.   *hyper-*

The antidote for quinidine and Pronestyl toxicity is _____ _____.   *sodium bicarbonate*

A common side effect associated with quinidine therapy is

_____.   *diarrhea*

30 *Nursing orders:* The patient receiving quinidine or Pronestyl
   1. When administering procaine amide intravenously, watch for
      the development of *(hypotension/hypertension)* and widening of   *hypotension*

      the _____ complex.   *QRS*

   2. *Remember:* Quinidine and Pronestyl are cardiac *(depressants/*   *depressants*
      stimulants). In toxic dosages they produce widening of the

      _____ complex. The antidote for quinidine and Pronestyl   *QRS*

      toxicity is _____ _____.   *sodium bicarbonate*
   3. Administer oral quinidine and Pronestyl with food or milk to
      decrease the incidence of gastrointestinal symptoms.

   With quinidine therapy, watch for the development of _____.   *diarrhea*

31 Diphenylhydantoin (Dilantin) acts by:
   1. depressing ectopic impulse formation in the atria, the A-V junc-
      tional tissue, and the ventricles
   2. accelerating A-V conduction
   Dilantin may be used in the management of acute and chronic ven-

   tricular _____.   *arrhythmias*
   This drug is also useful in the management of digitalis-induced arrhythmias, both *ventricular* and *supraventricular.*
   It is especially effective in the presence of a junctional tachycardia
   caused by digitalis toxicity.

32 In toxic dosages Dilantin can produce bradyarrhythmias and cardiac standstill. *Respiratory* depression can also be a toxic manifestation of Dilantin therapy. The degree of cardiac and respiratory
   depression produced appears to be related to the dose and speed
   of administration.
   Other *side effects* that may be associated with Dilantin therapy are
   visual disturbances and *gingivitis.*

33 *Let us review:* Dilantin acts by depressing ectopic impulse forma-

   tion and accelerating _____ conduction.   *A-V*
   Dilantin *(may/may not)* be used in the treatment of ventricular   *may*
   tachycardia.
   Dilantin *(may/may not)* be used in the treatment of arrhythmias   *may*

   associated with digitalis toxicity, especially _____ tachy- *junctional*
   cardia.
   When administering Dilantin, the nurse should observe for both

   respiratory and cardiac _____.   *depression*
   Other side effects associated with Dilantin are _____ disturbances *visual*

   and _____.   *gingivitis*

34 *Nursing orders:* The patient receiving Dilantin
   1. Infuse Dilantin intravenously with saline solutions, because
      Dilantin is incompatible with glucose solution. Use of a final fil-
      ter is recommended to further filter out incompatibilities not
      easily visible. Incompatibilities are still further avoided by IV
      push administration at a rate not to exceed 50 mg/min.

2. With intravenous administration, watch for the development of *bradyarrhythmias*, which may progress to _____ _____. Also observe for the development of *respiratory* _____.

3. Observe for disturbances in _____ and for _____.

cardiac
standstill
depression
vision   *gingivitis*

35 Propranolol (Inderal) may be used in the acute or long-term management of ventricular arrhythmias. Propranolol acts by depressing ectopic impulse formation in the _____.

ventricles

Note: Inderal also depresses impulse formation in the sinus node and decreases myocardial contractility. Because of these properties, Inderal is usually *not* the drug used in the initial management of ventricular arrhythmias in acute myocardial infarction.

Propranolol has other properties that allow it to be useful in the management of fast supraventricular arrhythmias. Therefore, a thorough discussion of this drug is presented beginning in frame 48.

36 Another drug that has been used in the management of certain ventricular arrhythmias is *Bretylium*. Bretylium has been used in the setting of acute myocardial infarction to *prevent* recurrent ventricular fibrillation by apparently raising the threshold for ventricular fibrillation.

Parasympathetic and sympathetic drugs

37 Before continuing our discussion of the pharmacological management of problems associated with acute myocardial infarction, it is necessary to discuss a classification of drugs that is based on the parasympathetic and sympathetic nervous systems. Certain parasympathetic and sympathetic drugs may be used in the pharmacological management of:
1. fast supraventricular arrhythmias
2. bradyarrhythmias
3. heart failure
4. shock

38 *Let us review:* The heart is richly innervated by both sympathetic and parasympathetic nerves.

Sympathetic fibers supply the _____ node, the _____, the _____ _____ tissue, and the _____ system.

S-A   *atria*   *A-V*
junctional; His-Purkinje

Parasympathetic fibers supply the _____ node, the _____ and the _____ _____ tissue.

S-A   *atria*
A-V junctional

Sympathetic stimulation *(increases/decreases)* the heart rate and *(accelerates/depresses)* A-V conduction.

Parasympathetic stimulation *(increases/decreases)* the heart rate and *(accelerates/depresses)* A-V conduction.

increases
accelerates
decreases
depresses

Certain chemicals in the body act as mediators and enable the parasympathetic and sympathetic nerves to have their characteristic effects.

The mediator of the sympathetic nervous system is *norepinephrine.*

The mediator of the parasympathetic nervous system is *acetylcholine.*

Certain drugs may *mimic* or *block* the effects of these chemical mediators.

39 The effects of sympathetic and parasympathetic stimulation on the heart may be classified as: (1) chronotropic—affecting heart rate; (2) dromotropic—affecting conduction through the A-V junctional tissue; and (3) inotropic—affecting contractility. When describing the responses of the heart to a drug, the terms *positive* and *negative* may be used with respect to these terms.

A drug that *increases* contractility has a *(positive/negative)* inotropic effect.

positive

A drug that *decreases* contractility has a *(positive/negative)* inotropic effect.

negative

40 Let us first consider drugs that mimic the *sympathetic nervous system*.

The sympathetic nervous system has two types of receptors: (1) alpha (α), and (2) beta (β).

Therefore, sympathetic drugs are classified into two groups: (1) alpha stimulators and alpha blockers, and (2) beta stimulators and beta blockers.

Alpha receptors are *primarily* located in the *peripheral blood vessels*.
Beta receptors are *primarily* located in the *heart* and *lungs*.

41 Let us first consider those drugs that stimulate the *beta* receptors.

Remember: Beta receptors are primarily located in the _____

heart

and _____.

lungs

Drugs that *stimulate* beta receptors, therefore, act on the _____

heart

and _____.

lungs

In the heart, beta stimulation produces:
1. a positive chronotropic effect
2. a positive dromotropic effect
3. a positive inotropic effect
4. increased ventricular automaticity

Therefore, it can be expected that beta stimulation will produce a(n) *(increased/decreased)* heart rate, *(accelerated/depressed)* A-V conduction, *(increased/decreased)* contractility, and increased

increased; accelerated
increased

ventricular _____.

automaticity

In the lungs beta stimulation causes *bronchodilation*.

42 Just as the beta receptors may be stimulated, they may also be *blocked*.

Drugs that *block* the beta receptors produce effects *opposite* from those of beta stimulators.

In the heart, beta blockers produce:
1. a *(positive/negative)* chronotropic effect
2. a *(positive/negative)* dromotropic effect
3. a *(positive/negative)* inotropic effect
4. *(increased/decreased)* ventricular automaticity

negative
negative
negative
decreased

Therefore, it can be expected that *beta blockers* will cause a(n) *(increased/decreased)* heart rate, *(accelerated/depressed)* A-V conduction, *(increased/decreased)* myocardial contractility, and de-

decreased; depressed
decreased

creased ventricular _____.

automaticity

In the lungs beta blockers cause bronchial *(dilation/constriction)*.

constriction

186

43 *Remember:* Alpha receptors are primarily located in the periph-

   eral _____ _____.   *blood vessels*
   Drugs that *stimulate* the alpha receptors, therefore, act on the pe-

   ripheral _____ _____. Alpha stimulation produces *vasocon-*   *blood vessels*
   striction.

44 Just as the alpha receptors may be stimulated, they may also be
   blocked. Drugs that *block* the alpha receptors produce an effect *op-*
   posite from that of the alpha stimulators.
   Therefore, alpha *blockers* produce *(dilation/constriction)* of the pe-   *dilation*
   ripheral blood vessels.

45 Let us now consider drugs that mimic the parasympathetic nervous
   system.
   Remember: Parasympathetic fibers supply the _____ node, the   *S-A*

   _____, and the A-V _____ tissue.   *atria   junctional*
   On the *heart,* parasympathetic stimulation produces:
   1. a negative chronotropic effect
   2. a negative dromotropic effect
   3. no effects on inotropy or ventricular automaticity
   Therefore, it can be expected that parasympathetic stimulation
   will cause a(n) *(increased/decreased)* heart rate and *(accelerated/*   *decreased*
   depressed) A-V conduction.   *depressed*
   Note: Parasympathetic stimulation produces no effects on inotropy
   or ventricular automaticity because there are no parasympathetic
   fibers in the ventricles.

46 Just as parasympathetic fibers may be stimulated, they may also
   be *blocked.*
   On the heart, parasympathetic *blockers* produce:
   1. a *(positive/negative)* chronotropic effect   *positive*
   2. a *(positive/negative)* dromotropic effect   *positive*
   Therefore, parasympathetic blockers will cause a(n) *(increased/*   *increased*
   decreased) heart rate and *(accelerated/depressed)* A-V conduction.   *accelerated*

The fast supraventricular arrhythmias

47 With this background, let us now consider the problem of fast *su-*
   praventricular arrhythmias.
   Remember: Initial therapy in the management of fast supraventricular arrhythmias is directed toward *(increasing/decreasing)*   *decreasing*
   the ventricular rate.
   Those drugs that are capable of decreasing the ventricular rate
   are: (1) beta blockers, and (2) parasympathetic stimulators.

Propranolol (Inderal)

48 An example of a pure beta blocking agent is propranolol (Inderal).
   Remember: Drugs that *block* the beta receptors of the sympathetic
   nervous system produce these effects on the heart and the lungs:
   1. decreased heart rate
   2. depressed A-V conduction
   3. decreased myocardial contractility perfusion
   4. depressed ventricular automaticity
   5. bronchoconstriction
   Inderal has the ability to *slow* A-V conduction. Therefore, it may
   be used in the therapy of fast supraventricular arrhythmias to

Check lungs for rale for CHF may develope wheezes   **187**

slow the ventricular rate. Inderal also has the ability to *(depress/*   *depress*
enhance) ventricular automaticity. Therefore, it may also be used

in the management of _____ arrhythmias.   *ventricular*

49 The effects of propranolol on A-V conduction, the heart rate, and
automaticity are therapeutic. However, the effect on the lungs is undesirable. The effect of propranolol on myocardial contractility is
undesirable in the setting of acute MI. However, because it has
the concurrent ability to reduce oxygen consumption as it depresses
contractility, propranolol has been used in the management of angina.
Inderal must be administered with caution to patients with severely
impaired myocardial function or hypotension and a history of
asthma or bronchospasm.
Propranolol is a *pure* beta blocker. Therefore, the exact antidote
for propranolol is a pure beta stimulator. Isoproterenol (Isuprel)
is an example of a pure beta stimulator. Atropine may also be used
as an antidote for Inderal.

50 *Let us review:* Propranolol is classified as a pure *(alpha/beta)*   *beta*

_____.   *blocker*
Therapeutic effects of propranolol include:
1. *(increased/decreased)* heart rate   *decreased*
2. *(accelerated/depressed)* A-V conduction   *depressed*
3. *(increased/decreased)* automaticity in the ventricles   *decreased*
Undesirable effects of propranolol are:
1. *(increased/decreased)* myocardial contractility   *decreased*
2. bronchial *(constriction/dilation)*   *constriction*
Note: Other beta blocking agents are available and may be selected
for use by some institutions. Practolol is a beta blocking agent that
is presently in common use outside the United States.

51 *Nursing orders:* The patient receiving propranolol
1. Have atropine or Isuprel at the bedside when giving IV.
2. Administer *with* caution in patients with:
— impaired myocardial function
— hypotension
— asthma
3. Administer *very slowly* when giving intravenously.
4. Check for *rales* and *wheezes* following administration.

Digitalis

52 An example of a drug that has some parasympathetic stimulating
properties is digitalis.
Remember: Drugs that stimulate the parasympathetic nervous system produce these effects on the heart: (1) *(increased/decreased)*   *decreased*
heart rate, and (2) *(accelerated/depressed)* A-V conduction.   *depressed*
Digitalis has the ability to slow A-V conduction and thus slow the
ventricular rate. Therefore, digitalis *may* be used in some settings
in therapy of fast supraventricular arrhythmias.

53 Another therapeutic effect of digitalis is its ability to *increase myocardial contractility.* Because of this property, digitalis is frequently indicated in the management of heart failure. The use of
digitalis in CHF will be considered in the section on the pharmacological management of CHF.

54 Undesirable effects of digitalis may also be seen. Digitalis has the ability to increase automaticity in the *atria, A-V junctional tissue,* and *ventricles.* In the presence of digitalis toxicity, this property may lead to the development of classic digitalis-induced arrhythmias.

1. PAT with block
2. nodal or junctional tachycardia
3. ventricular arrhythmias, especially ventricular bigeminy

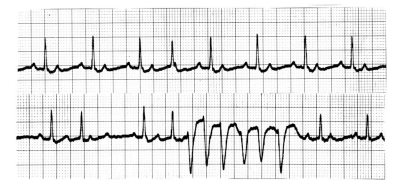

Fig. 8-1

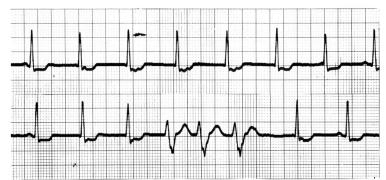

Other arrhythmias associated with digitalis toxicity are related to depressed automaticity in the sinus node and depressed conduction; for example, sinus bradycardia and A-V blocks.

Other signs of digitalis intolerance include symptoms such as anorexia, nausea, and vomiting.

Note: See frame 67 for the nursing orders for the patient receiving digitalis.

Note: Another parasympathetic stimulator that may be used in some settings to manage rapid supraventricular arrhythmias is *Tensilon.* Tensilon varies from digitalis in that it does not possess the additional properties of enhancing contractility and automaticity. It is a "purer" parasympathetic agent, more potent, and shorter in its duration of action.

The bradyarrhythmias

55 Let us now consider the problem of *bradyarrhythmias.*

Remember: The initial therapy in the management of bradyarrhythmias is directed toward increasing the _____ _____.   *ventricular rate*

The mechanisms by which the ventricular rate may be accelerated are:

1. increasing the sinus rate

2. accelerating A-V conduction
3. stimulating A-V junctional automaticity
4. stimulating ventricular automaticity

The drugs that are capable of increasing the ventricular rate are (1) the beta stimulators, and (3) the parasympathetic blockers.

Isoproterenol (Isuprel)

56 An example of a *pure beta stimulator* is isoproterenol (Isuprel).
Remember: Drugs that stimulate the beta receptors of the sympathetic nervous system produce these effects on the *heart* and *lungs:*
1. increased heart rate

2. accelerated _____ conduction   *A-V*

3. increased myocardial _____   *contractility*
4. increased A-V junctional automaticity

5. increased ventricular _____   *automaticity*
6. *(bronchoconstriction/bronchodilation)*   *bronchodilation*
Isuprel has the ability to *(increase/decrease)* the sinus rate, *(accel-*   *increase   accelerate*
erate/depress) A-V conduction, *(increase/decrease)* A-V junctional *increase*
automaticity and *(increase/decrease)* ventricular automaticity.   *increase*
Therefore it may be used in the management of *bradyarrhythmias.*
On the peripheral blood vessels, Isuprel acts as a *vasodilator.*
Note: The effects of Isuprel on BP will be discussed in the section on the pharmacological management of shock (see frames 75 and 76).

57 Because Isuprel has the ability to increase the heart rate and increase ventricular automaticity, there may be undesirable side effects of *tachyarrhythmias* and *ventricular* arrhythmias associated with its use.
Note: These side effects may also be observed when Isuprel is used

in respiratory therapy as a bronchial _____.   *dilator*

58 *Let us review:* Isuprel is classified as a pure *(alpha/beta)*   *beta*

_____. Therapeutic effects of Isuprel include: *stimulator*
1. *(increased/decreased)* heart rate   *increased*
2. *(accelerated/depressed)* A-V conduction   *accelerated*
3. *(increased/decreased)* myocardial contractility   *increased*
4. *(increased/decreased)* A-V junctional automaticity   *increased*
5. *(increased/decreased)* ventricular automaticity   *increased*
6. bronchial *(constriction/dilation)*   *dilation*
On the peripheral blood vessels, Isuprel acts as vaso-*(dilator/con-* *dilator*
strictor).
Note: See frame 77 for the nursing orders for the patient receiving Isuprel.

Atropine sulfate

59 An example of a drug that blocks the parasympathetic nervous system is *atropine.* The parasympathetic nerve that innervates the heart is the *vagus.* Therefore, atropine is also known as a *vagolytic* drug.
Remember: Drugs that block the parasympathetic nervous system have these effects on the heart: (1) *(increased/decreased)* heart   *increased*
rate, and (2) *(accelerated/depressed)* A-V conduction.   *accelerated*

190

Atropine has the ability to stimulate the sinus rate and accelerate A-V conduction and thus increase the ventricular rate.

Remember: Bradyarrhythmias may result in a symptomatic fall in cardiac output. In this setting acceleration of the ventricular rate *(is/is not)* indicated.

is

Recent studies indicate that caution be used when accelerating the heart rate in a recently injured ischemic myocardium.

Acceleration of the ventricular rate should be gradual, using small increments of atropine until patient symptoms disappear. Continued acceleration, even moderately, in this setting has been shown to increase oxygen consumption to the ischemic areas causing an unfavorable relation between myocardial oxygen supply and demand. A manifestation of this increase in oxygen consumption may be ventricular arrhythmias caused by ischemia.

60 Another undesirable effect of atropine is its ability to produce urinary retention. The bladder is innervated by parasympathetic fibers; thus blockage of these nerves may lead to difficulty in voiding in some patients.

Prolonged atropine therapy may cause mental confusion, which has been labelled "atropine madness" or "atropine psychosis."

Additional side effects associated with atropine therapy include: dryness of the mouth, flushing of the face, and dilation of the pupils.

Note: Atropine is contraindicated in patients with *glaucoma.*

61 *Let us review:* Atropine is classified as a *(parasympathetic/sympa-*   *parasympathetic*

thetic) _____.   *blocker*

Therapeutic effects of atropine include: (1) *(increased/decreased)*   *increased*
sinus rate, and (2) *(accelerated/depressed)* A-V conduction.   *accelerated*

Undesirable side effects of atropine include: (1) urinary _____,   *retention*

and (2) mental _____.   *confusion*
Other side effects associated with atropine include: (1) _____   *dryness*

of the mouth, (2) _____ of the face, and (3) _____   *flushing*   *dilation*
of the pupils.

62 *Nursing orders:* The patient receiving atropine
  1. Atropine is contraindicated in patients with _____.   *glaucoma*
  2. Monitor the heart rate when administering atropine for the therapeutic response.
  3. Watch for the development of urinary retention.
  4. With prolonged atropine therapy, watch for changes in sensorium.

DRUG THERAPY IN THE MANAGEMENT OF HEART FAILURE

63 Let us now discuss the pharmacological management of heart failure in the setting of acute myocardial infarction.

The major goals of pharmacological management of heart failure are: (1) to improve myocardial function, and (2) to decrease cardiac workload.

Digitalis

64 Let us first consider the use of drugs in improving myocardial function.

The primary drug used to improve myocardial contracility in heart failure is digitalis.

In therapeutic dosages, digitalis has these effects on the heart:
1. *(increased/decreased)* heart rate   *decreased*
2. *(accelerated/depressed)* A-V conduction   *depressed*
3. *(increased/decreased)* myocardial contractility   *increased*

Therefore, digitalis can be said to produce:
1. *(positive/negative)* chronotropic effect   *negative*
2. *(positive/negative)* dromotropic effect   *negative*
3. *(positive/negative)* inotropic effect   *positive*

Digitalis also has an effect on the ECG.

Remember: The electrolyte that affects contractility is _____.   *calcium*

Calcium affects the _____ segment on the ECG. The *effect* of digi-   *S-T*

talis on the ECG is to *shorten* the _____ segment. Digitalis also   *S-T*
causes shortening and sagging of the S-T segment.

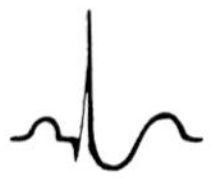

Fig. 8-2

DIGITALIS EFFECT

65 Digitalis is indicated in the management o*f heart failure* because
it has a *(positive/negative)* inotropic effect and thus *(increases/*   *positive; increases*
decreases) myocardial contractility.

Note: Any agent that has a positive inotropic effect also causes
increased oxygen consumption. Therefore, when there is already a
critical reduction in oxygen supply to the heart, digitalis must be
used with caution.

In the setting of acute myocardial infarction, digitalis may enhance
myocardial O_2 consumption and cause extension of the infarcted
area. The ischemic myocardium is also more sensitive to the effects
of digitalis toxicity. Thus digitalis is *not* the drug of choice in the
initial management of heart failure caused by MI. However, it is
often indicated in CHF caused by other mechanisms.

66 *Remember:* The undesirable side effects associated with digitalis
therapy are: (1) anorexia, (2) nausea and vomiting, and (3) arrhythmias—PAT with block, A-V junctional tachycardias, ventricular arrhythmias, A-V blocks, and sinus bradycardia.

67 *Nursing orders:* The patient receiving digitalis
   1. Observe for the therapeutic effects of digitalis:
      — Is heart failure improving?
      — Is the heart rate slowing?

Note: Digitalis may slow the heart rate simply by improving myocardial function.

   2. Observe for the development of anorexia.

Note: This is often the first sign of digitalis intolerance.

   3. Watch for the development of nausea and vomiting.
   4. Monitor the patient carefully for the development of arrhyth-
       mias:
      — PAT with block
      — junctional _____   *tachycardia*
      — ventricular arrhythmias—especially ventricular _____   *bigeminy*
      — sinus bradycardia
      — A-V block
   5. Check serum potassium (K^+) levels.

Remember: Hypokalemia potentiates the effects of digitalis.

6. Dilantin may be used in the management of digitalis-induced arrhythmias.

Diuretic agents

68 Let us now discuss the role of *diuretic agents* in the pharmacological management of heart failure.

One of the goals in the management of congestive heart failure is

to decrease cardiac _____.   *workload*

Diuretic agents accomplish this by decreasing the volume of fluid that must be pumped by the heart.

69 *Let us review:* In the presence of heart failure, events occur that lead to the accumulation of fluid.

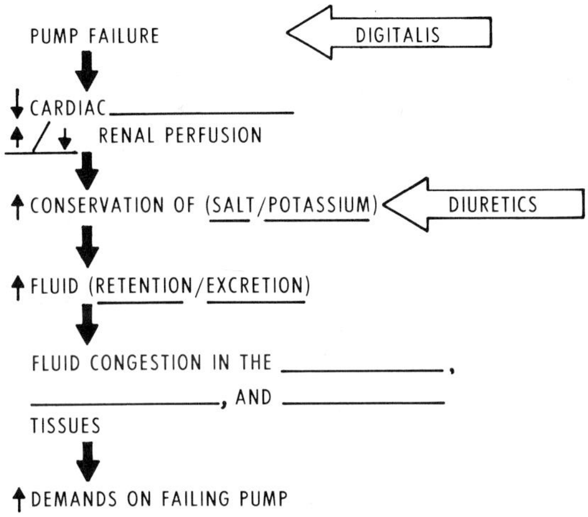

Fig. 8-3

output
decreased

salt

retention

lungs
liver   peripheral

This "vicious cycle" may be broken by correcting the underlying

flaw—the failing myocardium—with administration of _____.   *digitalis*

The disturbance of salt and water retention may be approached

by administering _____ agents.   *diuretic*

70 It appears that the common denominator of the action of commonly used diuretic agents is their ability to impair tubular reabsorption of *sodium.*

Remember: A major defect in congestive heart failure is the con-

servation of _____ and _____.   *sodium   water*

Reabsorption of sodium is blocked by (1) direct tubular action, and (2) inhibition of the hormones that regulate reabsorption.

Diuretics block the reabsorption of _____ and, therefore,   *sodium*

_____. In this way, fluid volume is *(increased/decreased)* and the   *water   decreased*
cardiac workload is *(increased/reduced)*.   *reduced*

71 The goals of diuretic therapy are:

1. to establish a negative balance of sodium and _____.   *water*
2. to correct any ECF volume *(overload/deficit)*   *overload*
3. to avoid volume and electrolyte disturbances

Any given diuretic agent has two major effects on the kidney: (1)

increases urine volume output, and (2) increases excretion of urine electrolytes.

72 There are complications associated with the use of diuretic agents:
1. hypovolemia and hypotension
2. electrolyte depletion, especially potassium
3. metabolic alkalosis

Diuretics cause a decrease in fluid volume, and thus have the potential for causing hypovolemic and hypotensive states.

Most diuretic agents also cause a loss of potassium. Therefore, diuresis may lead to the development of *(hypo-/hyper-)*kalemia.   *hypo-*

Remember: Chlorides (Cl⁻) are alos lost with the potassium (K⁺). When an anion (Cl⁻) is lost, the body attempts to compensate by

retaining another anion, _____ _____. This may   *bicarbonate (HCO₃⁻)*
eventually cause a metabolic *(acidosis/alkalosis).*   *alkalosis*

Potassium replacement solutions must also contain chlorides, if metabolic *(acidosis/alkalosis)* is to be avoided.   *alkalosis*

73 *Nursing orders:* The patient receiving diuretic agents
1. Observe for therapeutic effects following administration
— is there an increase in urine output?
— is heart failure improving?
2. Accurately record fluid intake and output.
3. Watch for the development of complications.
— hypovolemia and hypotension—assess hydration state
— hypokalemia—check serum potassium (K⁺) levels; is patient receiving K⁺ supplements?
— metabolic alkalosis—patients should be receiving supplements of *K⁻* and *Cl⁻*; check arterial pH and bicarbonate (HCO₃⁻) levels for evidence of alkalosis
4. Monitor daily serum electrolytes, BUN and creatinine.
5. With administration of furosemide (Lasix) and ethacrynic acid (Edecrin), watch for symptoms of ototoxicity (tinnitus, deafness).

DRUG THERAPY IN THE MANAGEMENT OF SHOCK

74 Let us now consider those drugs that may be used in the management of shock. (See Unit 7.)

Various sympathetic drugs have been used in the management of shock. The appropriate selection of sympathetic drugs to be used in cardiogenic shock is *highly* controversial and appears to be directly related to the cause of the shock and the ability of the *blood vessels* to respond to the drug.

75 *Remember:* Sympathetic drugs are classified into two groups: (1)

_____ ____ and (2) _____ ____.   *alpha (α)   beta (β)*
Alpha receptors are located *primarily* in the peripheral _____   *blood*

_____. Drugs that stimulate alpha receptors cause vaso-   *vessels*

_____. Drugs that block the alpha receptors cause vaso-   *constriction*

_____.   *dilatation*

Beta receptors are primarily found in the _____ and the _____.   *heart   lungs*
Drugs that stimulate beta receptors cause these effects on the heart:
1. increased _____ _____   *heart rate*

194

2. accelerated _____ _____   *A-V conduction*

3. increased _____ _____   *myocardial contractility*

4. increased ventricular _____   *automaticity*

Three major groups of drugs are currently used in the management of the shock state:

1. the myocardial stimulators—usually *(alpha/beta)* adrenergic agents   *beta*
2. the vasoconstrictor agents—usually *(alpha/beta)* adrenergic agents   *alpha*
3. the vasodilator agents

Isoproterenol (Isuprel)

76 A beta stimulating drug such as isoproterenol (Isuprel) may be indicated in *some* forms of shock.

BLOOD PRESSURE= | CARDIAC OUTPUT | × PERIPHERAL RESISTANCE

↑

ISUPREL ACTS HERE

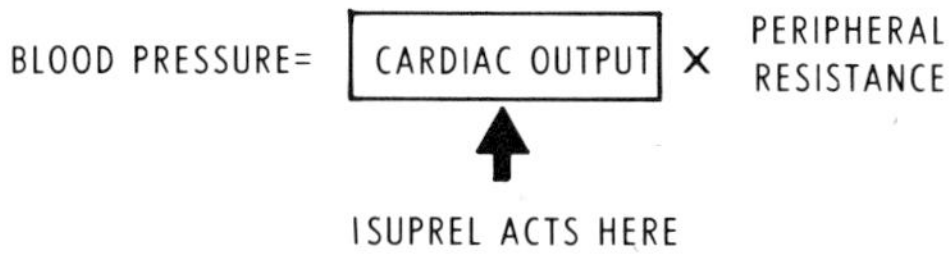

Fig. 8-4

Remember: Isuprel causes an *(increase/decrease)* in the heart rate and an *(increase/decrease)* in myocardial contractility.   *increase*
            increase

Thus cardiac output may be _____.   *increased*

Thus Isuprel will increase blood pressure directly, by influencing

_____ _____.   *cardiac output*

Isuprel, like other inotropic agents, also causes *increased oxygen consumption* by the *heart.* For this reason and its effect on electrical stability Isuprel is *not* indicated in cardiogenic shock resulting from coronary artery disease.

77 *Nursing orders:* The patient receiving Isuprel
1. Monitor blood pressure and cardiac status closely.
2. Watch for the development of tachyarrhythmias and ventricular arrhythmias with Isuprel.

Dopamine (Intropin)

78 A strong, primarily *inotropic* agent, such as dopamine (Intropin) may be indicated in some forms of shock as a myocardial stimulator in preference to Isuprel.

Remember: A positive *inotropic* agent increases myocardial

_____.   *contractility*

Dopamine, however, has the unique ability to selectively produce an increase in myocardial contractility without producing significant increases in rate or arrhythmia formation. Thus myocardial oxygen consumption is not as increased as it is with Isuprel.

79 Dopamine has the added *unique* ability to selectively produce vasoconstriction in some vessels and vasodilation in other vascular beds. Dopamine produces vasodilation in the renal, mesenteric, coronary, and intracerebral arterial beds.

Nursing orders: The patient receiving dopamine
1. Monitor blood pressure and cardiac status closely.
2. Watch urinary output for improvement.

Norepinephrine (Levophed) and metaraminol (Aramine)

80 Another group of drugs that may be used in the management of
some forms of shock are the *vasopressor drugs*. Drugs such as norepinephrine (Levophed), and metaraminol (Aramine), have both
alpha and *beta* properties. On the blood vessels they act as alpha
stimulators and cause *(vasoconstriction/vasodilation)*. On the heart   *vasoconstriction*
these drugs have some beta stimulating properties and cause a
slight positive *inotropic* effect.

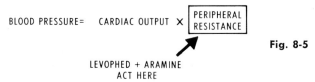

BLOOD PRESSURE=   CARDIAC OUTPUT   ×   PERIPHERAL
RESISTANCE

Fig. 8-5

LEVOPHED + ARAMINE
ACT HERE

81 Levophed and Aramine exhibit predominantly alpha adrenergic effects.
These drugs have been used in cardiogenic shock to support the
diastolic pressure and thus improve coronary perfusion. By elevat-
ing peripheral vascular resistance these drugs affect the heart's
afterload. By increasing afterload these drugs may *(enhance/re-*   *enhance*
duce) myocardial oxygen consumption.
Because these sympathomimetic drugs also have beta effects, they
have the potential for increasing oxygen consumption by affecting

heart rate and _____. They also have arrhythmogenic po-   *contractility*
tential.

82 *Nursing orders:* The patient receiving Levophed or Aramine
1. Monitor blood pressure and cardiac status closely.
— avoid sudden, severe increases in BP
— watch for the development of tachyarrhythmias and PVCs
2. Avoid infiltration into subcutaneous tissue; Levophed may
cause severe tissue sloughing.
Note: The antidote used to counteract the effects of Levophed on
the subcutaneous tissue is Regitine.
3. Patients receiving these drugs will probably have cold, clammy
skin. *Remember:* These drugs act as peripheral vasoconstrictors.

The vasodilators

83 Another group of drugs that are currently being used experimen-
tally in the management of refractory heart failure and cardiogenic
shock associated with coronary artery disease are the vasodilators.
The vasodilator presently in common use is sodium nitroprusside
(Nipride).

Sodium nitroprusside (Nipride)

84 *Remember:* Therapy in the management of coronary cardiogenic
shock is directed toward: (1) improving cardiac output, and (2)
improving myocardial oxygenation. This is accomplished by im-

proving coronary _____ _____ or reducing oxygen _____.   *blood flow; demands*
Sodium nitroprusside improves myocardial oxygenation by reduc-
ing oxygen demands.

85 *Remember:* Myocardial oxygen demands (oxygen consumption) are

dependent on the heart's: (1) rate, (2) _____, (3) _____,   *preload; afterload*
and (4) contractility.

86 Nitroprusside lowers *afterload* by producing arterial vasodilation. This reduction in arterial resistance reduces impedance to left ventricular emptying and thus *(increases/decreases)* cardiac output.   *increases*

87 Nitroprusside may reduce *preload* by producing venodilation. Venodilation results in a(n) *(increase/decrease)* in venous return,   *decrease*
which results in *(increased/decreased)* ventricular filling (preload).   *decreased*
When preload is reduced a(n) *(increase/decrease)* in LVEDP and   *decrease*
oxygen consumption occurs.

88 Although the effect of nitroprusside on preload is considered beneficial, the effect on afterload is thought to be most significant in contributing to the hemodynamic improvement seen during administration.

89 Nitroprusside should be administered only in intensive care units capable of hemodynamic monitoring. Factors such as pulmonary artery pressures, wedge pressures, arterial pressure, and cardiac output should be monitored.

90 *Nursing orders:* The patient receiving sodium nitroprusside (Nipride)
1. Hemodynamic parameters such as PA pressure, PCWP, arterial pressure, and cardiac output should be monitored during infusion.
2. Determine with the physician the "critical" LVEDP (wedge pressure) and arterial pressure to be achieved.
3. Prepare prescribed dose of Nipride.
   — mix only with dextrose in water
   — protect from deterioration by light by wrapping bottle in foil or other opaque material
   — infuse only with microdrip or similar type of device
   — follow manufacturer's suggestions regarding when drug should be discarded
   — do not add other medications to intravenous solutions containing Nipride
4. Monitor wedge pressure and arterial pressure frequently during infusion.
   — if pressure falls below determined critical levels, *immediately* slow Nipride infusion

Suggested readings

Amsterdam, E. A.: Cardiocirculatory effects of morphine sulfate: Mechanisms of action and therapeutic application, Heart Lung 3(3):495, May-June 1974.

Amsterdam, E. A., Massumi, R., Zelis, R., and Mason, D. T.: Evaluation and management of cardiogenic shock. Part II. Drug therapy, Heart Lung 1(5):663, Sept.-Oct. 1972.

Amsterdam, E. A., and others: The use of diuretics in acute myocardial infarction, Heart Lung 2(3):434, May-June 1973.

Bigger, J. T., Jr., and Heissenbuttle, R. N.: The use of procaine amide and Lidocaine in the treatment of cardiac arrhythmias. In Friedberg, C. K., editor: Current status of drugs in cardiovascular disease, New York, 1969, Grune & Stratton, Inc.

Cannon, P. J., and Kilcoyrea, M. M.: Ethacrynic acid and furosemide; renal pharmacology and clinical use. In Friedberg, C. K., editor: Current status of drugs in cardiovascular disease, New York, 1969, Grune & Stratton, Inc.

Castellanos, A., Ghafour, A. A., and Soffer, A.: Digitalis-induced arrhythmias; recognition and therapy, Cardiov. Ther. 1:108, 1970.

Castellanos, A., Lemberg, L., and Centurion, M. J.: The mechanisms of digitalis-induced ventricular fibrillation, Dis. Chest 54:53, 1968.

Cohn, J. N.: Vasodilator therapy of myocardial infarction (editorial), New Engl. J. Med., June 20, 1974.

Conn, H. S., editor: Current therapy 1971, Philadelphia, 1971, W. B. Saunders Co.

Damato, A. N.: Diphenylhydantoin; pharmacological and clincal use. In Friedberg, C. K., editor: Current status of drugs in cardiovascular disease, New York, 1969, Grune & Stratton, Inc.

Damato, A. N., and others: The effect of diphenylhydantoin on atrioventricular and intraventricular conduction in man, Am. Heart J. 79: 51-56, 1970.

Driefus, L. S., and Watanabe, Y.: Current status of diphenylhydantoin, Am. Heart J. 79:709-713, 1970.

Epstein, S. E., Redwood, D. R., and Smith, E. R.: Atropine and acute myocardial infarction, Circulation 45:1273, June 1972.

Franciosa, J. A., and others: Improved left ventricular function during nitroprusside infusion in acute myocardial infarction, Lancet, Mar. 25, 1972.

Gibson, D., and Sowton, E.: The use of beta-adrenergic receptor blocking drugs in dysrhythmias. In Friedberg, C. K., editor: Current status of drugs in cardiovascular disease, New York, 1969, Grune & Stratton, Inc.

Goldberg, L.: Dopamine—clinical uses of an endogenous catecholamine, New Engl. J. Med. 291 (14):707.

Goodman, L. L., and Gilman, A.: The pharmacological basis of therapeutics, London, 1969, The Macmillan Co.

Goodman, L. L., and Gilman, A.: The pharmacological basis of therapeutics, New York, 1970, The Macmillan Co.

Greenblatt, D. J., and Shader, R.: Drug therapy: Anticholinergics, New Engl. J. Med. 288(23): 1215, June 7, 1973.

Guia, N. H.: Treatment of refractory heart failure of infusion of nitroprusside, New Engl. J. Med. 291(12):587, Sept. 19, 1974.

Heissenbuttle, R. N., and Bigger, J. T., Jr.: Effect of oral quinidine with changes in QRS duration, Am. Heart J. 79:453-462, 1970.

Kim, K. E., and others: Ethacrynic acid and furosemide; diuretic and hemodynamic effects and clinical uses, Am. J. Cardiol. 27:407-416, 1971.

Kleit, S. A., and others: Diuretic therapy—current status, Am. Heart J. 79:700, 1970.

Knoebel, S. B., and Rasmussen, S.: Myocardial blood flow: Newer clinical considerations, Heart Lung 3(1):78, Jan.-Feb. 1974.

Lemberg, L., and others: Cardiac drugs in the coronary care unit, Chest 59:289, 1971.

Lown, B., Garrison, H., and others: Sensitivity to digitalis drugs in acute myocardial infarction, Am. J. Cardiol. Vol. 30, Sept. 1972.

McAllister, R. G., Jr.: The possible role of antiarrhythmic drugs in the prevention of sudden death, Heart Lung 2(6):857, 1973.

Miller, R. R., and others: Procaineamide: Reappraisal of an old antiarrhythmic drug, Heart Lung 2(2):277, Mar.-Apr. 1973.

Misra, S. N., and others: Hemodynamic effects of adrenergic stimulating and blocking agents in cardiogenic shock and low output state after myocardial infarction, Am. J. Cardiol. 31:6, June 1973.

Noble, R. J., Dickerson, L. S., and Fisch, C.: The use and abuse of digitalis in acute myocardial infarction, Heart Lung 1(6):762, Nov.-Dec. 1972.

Selzer, A.: The use and abuse of quinidine, Heart Lung 1(6):755, Nov.-Dec. 1972.

Singer, D. H., and Geneick, R. E.: Pharmacology of cardiac arrhythmias. In Friedberg, C. F., editor: Current status of drugs in cardiovascular disease, New York, 1969, Grune & Stratton, Inc.

Surawicz, B., and Lasseter, K. C.: Effects of drugs on the electrocardiogram, Prog. Cardiov. Dis. 8(1):26, July 1970.

Vismara, L. A., Mason, D. T., and Amsterdam, E. A.: Cardiocirculatory effects of morphine sulfate: Mechanisms of action and therapeutic application, Heart Lung 3(3):495, May-June 1974.

Electrical intervention in acute myocardial infarction

Electrical intervention in the management of cardiac arrhythmias consists of either *countershock* or *pacemakers*.

COUNTERSHOCK

1 Let us first consider *countershock*.

Countershock is the delivery of a high intensity charge to the heart that results in complete depolarization of the myocardium. This charge has the potential for interrupting certain arrhythmias and thus allows the normal pacemaker, the S-A node, to resume control of the rhythm.

Note: If the S-A node is depressed, it may not resume control of the rhythm. If this occurs, lower centers having the property of automaticity may assume control of the rhythm, or total electrical failure may occur.

There are two types of countershock: (1) cardioversion and (2) defibrillation.

Definitions

2 *Cardioversion* refers to the delivery of a *synchronized* charge to the myocardium. *Synchronization* means that the countershock machine is programmed to deliver its charge *only* after "sensing" the patient's major QRS deflection.

3 The term *synchronization*, therefore, implies that there is a(n)

_____ mechanism.   *sensing*

A synchronized charge will be released *only* after the machine

"senses" the major _____ deflection.   *QRS*

The charge is then released *during* the QRS phase of the cardiac cycle.

A synchronized charge *(will/will not)* be delivered during the T   *will not*
wave.

A synchronized charge *(will/will not)* cause ventricular fibrillation.   *will not*

4 *Cardioversion* is used in the management of fast arrhythmias when a QRS complex is present.

Therefore, cardioversion *(may/may not)* be used in the manage-   *may*
ment of atrial fibrillation with a rapid ventricular response.

Cardioversion *(may/may not)* be used in the management of ven-   *may*
tricular tachycardia.

Cardioversion *(may/may not)* be used in the management of ven-   *may not*
tricular fibrillation.

5 The other form of countershock is *defibrillation*.

Defibrillation refers to the delivery of a *nonsynchronized* charge to the myocardium. The term *nonsynchronized* implies that there *(is/*
is not) a sensing mechanism.   *is not*

6 A *nonsynchronized* charge is indicated *only* for fast arrhythmias where there is no QRS complex present.

The only fast arrhythmia in which there is *no* QRS complex present is _____ _____. *ventricular fibrillation*

Therefore, defibrillation is used only in the treatment of

_____ _____. *ventricular fibrillation*

Defibrillation *(may/may not)* be used in the management of atrial fibrillation with a rapid ventricular response. *may not*

In ventricular fibrillation there *(is/is not)* a QRS complex present. *is not*

A *synchronized* charge, then, *(would/would not)* fire during VF. *would not*

An unsynchronized charge, however, *(will/will not)* fire during VF. *will*

7 *Note:* Another form of unsynchronized shock may be delivered by a blow to the precordium. This mechanical shock, although of low intensity, can also result in complete depolarization of the myocardium and can terminate certain arrhythmias.

8 The amount of electrical voltage required for the delivery of countershock is dependent upon the characteristics of the arrhythmia. *Note:* The countershock charge is registered in watt/seconds.

9 *Supraventricular arrhythmias generally* require smaller amounts of charge to be abolished, such as 10 to 100 watt/seconds.

Ventricular tachycardia may be abolished with the same voltage. However, because of its rapid disintegration into VF, larger amounts of voltage may be required, even up to 400 watt/seconds.

Ventricular fibrillation represents the most deteriorated electrical activity. Therefore, it usually requires the highest voltage to be abolished—400 watt/seconds.

10 *Remember:* Cardioversion and defibrillation differ in these ways:
1. synchronized vs. nonsynchronized charge
2. degree of voltage required
3. indications (absence or presence of a QRS complex)

11 *Let us review:* Cardioversion is used in the management of *(fast/* *fast*

slow) arrhythmias when there is still a _____ complex present. *QRS*

Cardioversion is the delivery of a(n) *(synchronized/unsynchronized)* charge to the myocardium. *synchronized*

The term *synchronized* implies that there *(is/is not)* a *sensing* mechanism. *is*

A synchronized charge will always be delivered during the _____ *QRS*

_____. *complex*

Synchronization may be used in all fast arrhythmias, except

_____ _____. *ventricular fibrillation*

Defibrillation is the delivery of a(n) *(synchronized/unsynchronized)* charge. *unsynchronized*

Another form of unsynchronized shock is the _____ *precordial*

_____. *blow*

An electrical charge will abolish arrhythmias by causing complete

myocardial _____. *depolarization*

12 The mechanical equipment necessary for cardioversion and defibrillation is:
1. a power generator, which builds up the charge

200

2. a set of paddles to deliver the charge
3. a monitor scope or ECG write-off to document the ECG patterns

Preparation for countershock

13 There are common principles that must be considered prior to the delivery of countershock.

Following the delivery of a countershock charge to the myocardium, there is always a period of *electrical instability,* which may result in arrhythmias. Therefore, any factors that enhance electrical instability should be managed prior to the delivery of the charge, if possible. The following have been identified as factors that enhance electrical instability:
1. hypokalemia
2. hypoxia
3. digitalization
4. acidosis or alkalosis

14 Following countershock, there will be a period of _____ _____.

Electrical instability is enhanced in the presence of _____, _____, _____, and _____ or _____.

Countershock in the presence of these abnormalities may result in _____.

electrical instability
hypokalemia

hypoxia; digitalis; acidosis; alkalosis

arrhythmias

15 *Nursing orders:*
1. Check serum K^+ levels prior to cardioversion.
2. Assess respiratory status via arterial blood gas analysis (Po_2 levels), auscultation of the lungs, and observation of rate and character of respirations.
3. If the patient is digitalized:
   — know when last dose was given
   — know cumulative total of digitalis administered
4. Check acid-base balance via arterial blood gas analysis (pH, Pco_2, HCO_3 levels).
5. Anticipate ventricular arrhythmias postcardioversion: have Xylocaine at bedside.

Note: These orders are especially indicated in the setting of elective cardioversion.

16 Another factor to be considered is *premedication,* which is required if countershock is an elective procedure. Two drugs commonly used in this setting are: (1) diazepam (Valium) and (2) sodium methohexital (Brevital). Other short-acting barbiturates have also been used.

Note: These drugs are primarily used for their transient amnesic effect rather than for general anesthesia.

17 Respiratory depression and hypoventilation can occur following the administration of either of these drugs. Hypoventilation can then lead to hypoxia and respiratory acidosis.

Remember: Hypoxia and acidosis can *(increase/decrease)* electrical instability.

increase

The major side effect associated with the intravenous administration of Valium and Brevital is _____ _____.

respiratory depression

Respiratory depression results in _____, which

hypoventilation

201

can lead to the development of _____ and _____.   *hypoxia*   *acidosis*

18 *Nursing orders:*
1. Patient must have a patent and stable intravenous line.
2. Watch for hypoventilation.
3. Have an Ambu bag, airway, and supplementary oxygen at the bedside.
4. Patient should be stimulated and encouraged to breathe deeply and cough following the cardioversion.
5. Provide for physical safety until patient has recovered from the effects of the drugs.
6. Be aware that paradoxical reactions may be seen following intravenous administration of Valium (irritability, hyperactive behavior, confusion).

19 Other factors to be considered are related to the *preparation* of the *patient,* preparation of the *equipment,* and *monitoring* and *safety* aspects.

20 *Nursing orders:*
1. Explain the procedure to the patient; avoid use of frightening terms such as *electric* and *shock* when describing the procedure.
   — patient should be aware that the procedure will make his heart slower and more regular and will relieve his symptoms
   — some patients may benefit by observing pre- and postcardioversion strips of their rhythm
   — the cardioversion procedure may be described as being analogous to a "message" delivered to the heart
2. Place the patient in a supine position, if possible.
3. Remove dentures.
4. Securely attach electrodes and obtain clear ECG trace with no artifact.

21 5. Check for synchronization, if required.
6. Charge machine to desired voltage.
7. Apply conductive paste to paddles.
8. Position paddles correctly.
Note: In the setting of elective cardioversion, *anteroposterior* paddles are usually preferred, since a discharge directly through the heart is usually more effective. Paddles are also designed to be placed on the precordium in a *transverse* position.
In emergency settings, *transverse* paddles are usually preferred, because one person can apply them rapidly. The correct positioning for both types of paddles is presented in Fig. 9-1.
9. Apply paddles firmly to chest wall.

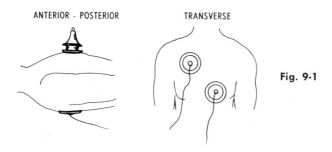

ANTERIOR - POSTERIOR   TRANSVERSE

Fig. 9-1

22 10. Before delivering the charge, make certain that no one is in

contact with the bed or patient, and avoid contact with wet areas that may conduct the current.

11. After delivery of the charge, immediately evaluate the rhythm and corresponding mechanical activity by checking for pulses; subsequent shocks may be necessary if the arrhythmia is not abolished.

Note: Failure of a properly delivered high intensity charge to convert the arrhythmia may indicate the presence of a secondary problem such as *hypoxia, acidosis* or *alkalosis,* or *drug toxicity.*

12. Following the delivery of the charge, continue monitoring to observe for development or recurrence of arrhythmias.

13. In patients who have had long-standing atrial fibrillation, observe for signs of embolism to brain, lung, or extremities after cardioversion.

PACEMAKERS

23 *Remember:* Electrical intervention in the management of cardiac

arrhythmias consists of either *countershock* or _____.   *pacemakers*
Let us now discuss *pacemakers.*
The function of a cardiac pacemaker is to provide an artificial electrical stimulus when the heart's own electrical system is failing.

24 *Remember:* The heart has an intrinsic electrical system that allows for the *origination* and *conduction* of electrical energy. When the heart's electrical system is failing, there will be disturbances in these *electrical* properties. The most significant manifestations of

this failure are *bradyarrhythmias,* or *(slow/fast) rates.*   *slow*
Therefore, pacemakers are used primarily in the management of

_____ _____.   *slow rates*

25 *Let us review:* Electrical failure may result from disturbances in

the ability of the heart to _____ and/or _____ elec-   *originate   conduct*
trical impulses.
The most significant manifestation of this electrical failure is

_____, or _____ rates.   *bradyarrhythmias; slow*
The device that is used in the management of slow rates secondary

to electrical failure is known as a _____.   *pacemaker*

26 An artificial pacemaker consists of two essential components: a *pulse generator,* which acts as an energy source for the stimulus, and a *catheter* to deliver the electrical stimulus. Some temporary pacing units also utilize a *bridging cable* as an extension between the energy source and the catheter.

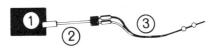

Fig. 9-2

1. Pulse generator
2. Bridging table
3. Catheter

27 When the pacemaker stimulus is delivered, a sharp, narrow deflection is seen on the ECG. This is known as the *stimulus artifact* or *pacing spike.*

The pacemaker stimulus is seen on the ECG as a pacing _____.   *spike*

28 The heart will respond to a pacemaker stimulus because it has the property of *excitability*.
Remember: Excitability is defined as the ability of the heart to respond to an electrical _____.   *stimulus*

29 Pacemakers may be utilized on a *temporary* or *permanent* basis, depending upon the clinical setting.
The pulse generators of *permanent* pacemakers may be implanted and the catheter positioned in contact with either the endocardium or epicardium.
Temporary pacemakers use an external energy source. The pacing catheter is threaded transvenously into the right side of the heart so that contact is established with the *(endocardium/epicardium)*.   *endocardium*

30 The principles of pacing are similar for both _____ and   *permanent*
_____ pacemakers. However, the temporary transvenous   *temporary*
pacemaker will be emphasized here, for it is used most commonly in the setting of acute MI.

Classification of pacemakers

31 Pacemakers are classified according to their *location* and *mode of action*.
Classification according to *location* is dependent upon the site of the stimulating, or pacing, electrodes.

32 Although the battery pack within the pulse generator creates and releases the electricity, the stimulus is delivered from *electrodes*, which are located on the *catheter*.
The release of the stimulus appears on the ECG as a *pacing spike*. The interval between the spikes of two consecutively paced beats is the *automatic interval*. This interval should approximately correspond to the rate at which the pacemaker is set to automatically fire.
This interval should be measured to confirm that stimuli are being released at the prescribed automatic rate.
The rate at which the pacemaker is releasing stimuli is known as the _____ interval.   *automatic*

33 The stimuli are released via _____, which are located on the   *electrodes*
catheter tip. These electrodes are referred to as the stimulating or pacing electrodes.
When the stimulating electrodes are located in the ventricles, the pacemaker is classified as a(n) _____ pacemaker.   *ventricular*
When the stimulating electrodes are located in the atria, the pacemaker is classified as _____.   *atrial*

34 The *modes of pacing* used in the setting of coronary care are:
1. continuous
2. inhibited (demand)
3. triggered (synchronized)
4. sequential (bifocal demand)
The modes of pacing are differentiated by the presence and/or function of a *sensing* mechanism. A sensing mechanism interprets in-

204

formation which is received about the patient's own rhythm. The sensing mechanism thus allows the pacemaker to be "sensitive" to the patient's own rhythm.

If the sensing electrodes are located in the atrium, the pacemaker senses the patient's _____ _____. If the sensing electrodes are located in the ventricle, the pacemaker senses the patient's _____ _____.

P waves

QRS complexes

35 The *continuous* pacemaker fires continuously without regard for the patient's own rhythm. It, therefore, *(is/is not)* sensitive to the patient's own rhythm and *(does/does not)* have a sensing mechanism. The three other modes of pacing all have sensing mechanisms but their sensing *functions* differ.

is not
does not

36 In the *inhibited* mode, the sensing mechanism allows the pacing spike to be *inhibited* in the presence of the patient's own rhythm. Therefore, the pacemaker fires only when needed or on *demand*. For this reason, the inhibited mode of pacing is referred to as true _____ pacing.

In the *triggered* mode the sensing mechanism determines when or not the pacing spike is released.

In the *sequential* mode the sensing mechanism controls *two* spikes firing in sequence.

demand

37 In all pacemakers with a *sensing* mechanism there is an escape interval. The interval is *reset* each time an impulse is sensed. If no natural impulse occurs before the set time interval, the pacemaker *(will/will not)* escape and fire.

The duration of the escape interval in most pacemakers approximately corresponds to the rate at which the pacemaker usually releases its impulses, or the _____ interval. For example, if the automatic interval is 1 second (corresponding to a rate of 60) and the patient's rate falls below 75, the pacemaker will escape and fire at a rate of _____.

Thus the escape interval ensures that the patient's heart rate will never fall below a certain minimal rate.

will

automatic

60

38 *Let us review:* Pacemakers are classified according to _____ and _____ of _____.

Classification according to location is dependent upon the site of the _____, or pacing, electrodes.

Classification according to mode of action depends upon the presence and/or function of the _____ mechanism.

The interval between two consecutive pacing spikes is known as the _____ interval.

The interval between a natural impulse and the next automatically paced beat is known as the _____ interval.

location

mode   *action*

stimulating

sensing

automatic

escape

Atrial pacemakers

39 Let us now examine both the location and mode of action of some commonly used pacemakers:

A pacemaker with *stimulating* electrodes in the atrium is classi-

fied as a(n) _____ pacemaker.   *atrial*

Remember: When a pacemaker fires, the electrical stimulus that

appears on the ECG is known as a(n) _____ _____.   *pacing spike*

When a pacemaker is stimulating the *atrium,* it can be expected

that each pacing spike will produce a(n) _____ wave.   *P*

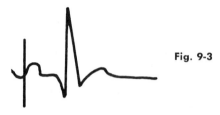

Fig. 9-3

40 The only mode of atrial pacing currently being used in the setting
of acute MI is the *continuous atrial pacemaker.*

Remember: Pacemakers are classified according to _____   *location*

and _____ ____ _____.   *mode of action*

Continuous refers to the *mode of action* and *atrial* refers to the
location of the stimulating electrodes.

41 A *continuous* pacemaker *is not* sensitive to the patient's own
rhythm. The continuous atrial pacemaker, therefore, *(does/does*   *does not*
not) have a sensing mechanism.

42 The catheter of the continuous atrial pacemaker is usually threaded
transvenously into the *(right/left)* atrium. It essentially bypasses   *right*
the S-A node and acts as an artificial *S-A node.* It is used *only* in
the presence of a healthy and normally functioning A-V node.

43 Continuous atrial pacemakers *(should/should not)* be used in the   *should not*
presence of A-V block. Continuous atrial pacemakers *(may/may*   *may*
not),* however, be used in the setting of sinus block or sinus arrest.

44 The continuous atrial pacemaker is also used in the treatment of
ventricular arrhythmias that are associated with *slow rates.*
In this setting, the pacemaker is used to *drive* the heart at a rate
(faster/slower) than the patient's own rate. This concept is known   *faster*
as *electrical overdrive.*
Note: Electrical overdrive is employed only when pharmacological
overdrive is ineffective or unsafe.

45 *Let us review:* The continuous atrial pacemaker acts as an artifi-

cial _____ node.   *S-A*

The continuous atrial pacemaker may be used only when conduc-

tion through the _____ node is normal.   *A-V*

When a pacemaker is stimulating the atrium, each pacing spike

should produce a(n) _____ _____.   *P wave*

	CLASSIFICATION	COMPLEX FOLLOWING SPIKE	LOCATION	MODE OF ACTION	INDICATIONS
A	ATRIAL CONTINUOUS	P WAVE	ATRIA	CONTINUOUS	1. SINUS ARREST 2 S-A BLOCK 3. ELECTRICAL OVERDRIVE

Fig. 9-4

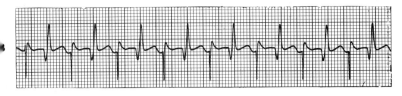

Ventricular pacemakers

47 A pacemaker with stimulating electrodes in the ventricles is classi-

fied as a(n) _____ pacemaker.   *ventricular*

When a pacemaker is stimulating the ventricles, each pacing spike

should produce a(n) _____ _____.   *QRS complex*
In ventricular pacing, the impulse is originating in the _____.   *ventricles*
Therefore, it can be expected that the QRS complex will be *(wide/*   *wide*
narrow)*.

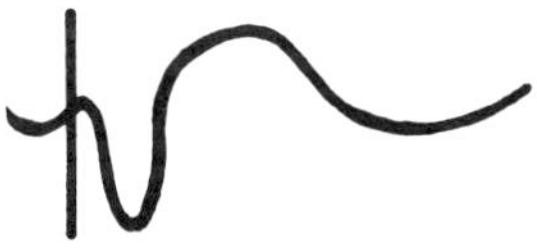

Fig. 9-5

The most common type of pacing used in the setting of acute MI is
ventricular pacing.

Continuous ventricular pacemaker

48 The earliest mode of ventricular pacing developed was the continuous. The continuous ventricular pacemaker is *not* sensitive to the
patient's own rhythm. Therefore, it *(does/does not)* have a sensing   *does not*
mechanism.

The continuous ventricular pacemaker fires continuously *(with/*
without)* regard for the patient's own beats.   *without*

49 A pacing spike, therefore, *(could/could not)* fall during the vul- *could*

nerable phase of the cardiac cycle and cause _____ _____.   *repetitive firing*
Because of this danger, the continuous mode of ventricular pacing
is no longer being used in the setting of acute MI.

	CLASSIFICATION	COMPLEX FOLLOWING SPIKE	LOCATION	MODE OF ACTION	INDICATION
A	CONTINUOUS VENTRICULAR	QRS COMPLEX	VENTRICLES	CONTINUOUS	A-V BLOCK

Fig. 9-6

B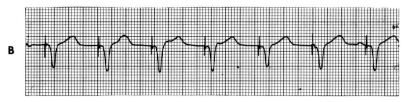

QRS-inhibited (demand) ventricular pacemaker

51 The mode of pacing being used most frequently in the setting of coronary care at the present time is the *QRS-inhibited ventricular pacemaker.*

This pacemaker has both a *stimulating* and a *sensing* mechanism. Both stimulating and sensing are accomplished via electrodes located in the ventricles.

This pacemaker is classified as *ventricular* because the *stimulating*

electrodes are located in the _____.   *ventricles*

52 The *sensing* electrodes are located in the ventricles. Thus the pacemaker will be "sensitive" to the patient's _____ _____.   *QRS complex*

Each time the patient has his own QRS complex, this information is transmitted back to the pacemaker. This pacemaker is programmed to *not* fire when the patient has his own QRS complex. The pacemaker stimulus is *inhibited* by the patient's own QRS complex. Thus the name *QRS-inhibited* ventricular pacemaker was derived.

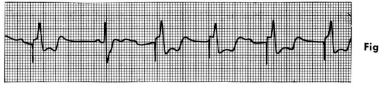

Fig. 9-7

53 Like all pacemakers with a sensing mechanism the QRS-inhibited pacemaker has an escape interval. The escape interval approximately corresponds to the automatic interval, or the rate at which the pacemaker is set to fire. If the pacemaker is set at a rate of 75 beats per minute and the patient's own rate falls below 75, the pacemaker *(will/will not)* fire. This pacemaker fires only when needed,   *will*

or *on demand.* For this reason, the QRS-inhibited ventricular pacemaker is commonly referred to as the *demand* ventricular pacemaker.

54 The *QRS-inhibited* (demand) *ventricular pacemaker* is ideal for

208

use in the setting of acute myocardial infarction because of its two unique characteristics:
1. inhibition in the presence of the patient's own QRS complex
2. ability to fire only when needed, or *on demand*

55 IN SUMMARY:

A

CLASSIFICATION	COMPLEX FOLLOWING SPIKE	LOCATION	MODE OF ACTION	INDICATIONS
QRS INHIBITED VENTRICULAR (DEMAND)	QRS COMPLEX	VENTRICLES	DEMAND	1. A-V BLOCK 2. ELECTRICAL OVERDRIVE

Fig. 9-8

B

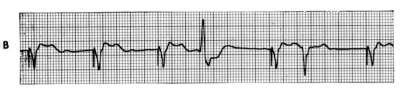

QRS-triggered (synchronized) ventricular pacemaker

56 Another mode of ventricular pacing used in some institutions following acute MI is the *QRS-triggered ventricular pacemaker.*
Like the QRS-inhibited pacemaker, the QRS-triggered ventricular pacemaker has both a *stimulating* and a *sensing* mechanism. Both stimulating and sensing are accomplished via electrodes located in the right ventricle.

57 These two modes of pacemakers are also alike in their ability to fire when the patient's own rate falls below a preset limit.

58 These two pacemakers differ in the way they are programmed to respond to the information that is transmitted about the QRS complex.
Remember: The QRS-inhibited pacemaker *(does/does not)* fire when the patient has his own QRS.

does not

59 *The QRS-triggered* pacemaker, however, *does* fire when the patient has his own QRS. The pacing spike is seen in the *middle* of the QRS complex. The patient's own QRS, then, *triggers* the pacing spike. Thus the name *QRS-triggered* pacemaker was derived. This pacemaker is also referred to as the *synchronized ventricular pacemaker.*
Note: The spike in the middle of the patient's own QRS complex indicates that the sensing mechanism is functioning normally. The spike does alter QRS morphology and thus may interfere with the evaluation of the ventricular complex. This introduces a potential problem in interpretation of certain arrhythmias.

60 *Let us review:* The QRS-triggered ventricular pacemaker *stimulates* and *senses* via electrodes in the _____.

ventricles

The pacemaker fires each time the patient has his own _____

QRS

_____.

complex

If the patient's own rate falls below a preset limit, the QRS-trig-

209

gered pacemaker *(will/will not)* fire and pace the _____.   *will*   *ventricles*
The QRS-triggered pacemaker *(may/may not)* be used in the pres-   *may*
ence of A-V block.

61 IN SUMMARY:

A

CLASSIFICATION	COMPLEX FOLLOWING SPIKE	LOCATION	MODE OF ACTION	INDICATION
QRS-TRIGGERED VENTRICULAR (SYNCHRONIZED)	QRS COMPLEX	VENTRICLES	TRIGGERED	A-V BLOCK

Fig. 9-9

B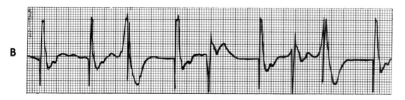

P wave–triggered (synchronized) ventricular pacemaker

62 The P wave–triggered ventricular pacemaker has both a stimulating and a sensing mechanism.
In this mode of pacing, two catheters are utilized—one in the atrium
and one in the ventricle.
The pacing, or stimulating, electrodes are located in the *ventricles.*

Thus this pacemaker is classified as _____.   *ventricular*
The sensing electrodes, however, are located in the *atrium.* Thus

this pacemaker is sensitive to the patient's _____ _____.   *P waves*

63 In this mode of pacing the P wave *triggers* the firing of the ventric-

ular pacemaker. Thus the name *P wave*–_____ ventricu-   *triggered*
lar pacemaker was derived.
Note: This pacemaker is also known as the atrial *synchronized* ventricular pacemaker.

64 This pacemaker essentially bypasses the A-V node and acts as an

artificial _____ node. It, therefore, *(may/may not)* be used in the   *A-V*   *may*
management of A-V block.

65 Like all pacemakers with a sensing mechanism the P wave–triggered ventricular pacemaker has an escape interval. If after a set
interval a P wave fails to occur, the ventricular pacemaker will escape and fire. If the atrial rate exceeds a certain limit the ventricular pacemaker will fire independently at a fixed rate.
Note: Because this mode of pacing is most frequently used in the
setting of chronic A-V block in children, it is not discussed in detail in this text.

	CLASSIFICATION	COMPLEX FOLLOWING SPIKE	LOCATION	MODE OF ACTION	INDICATION
A	P WAVE TRIGGERED (SYNCHRONIZED) VENTRICULAR	QRS COMPLEX	VENTRICLE	TRIGGERED	CHRONIC A-V BLOCK IN CHILDREN

Fig. 9-10

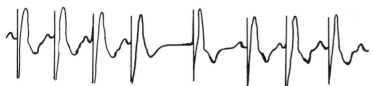

Sequential (bifocal demand) pacemaker

67 The latest mode of pacing developed for use in the setting of acute MI is the *sequential pacemaker*.
The sequential pacemaker is classified as *both* an *atrial* and a *ventricular* pacemaker because it has stimulating electrodes in *both*

the _____ and the _____.   *atrium   ventricles*

68 In this mode of pacing *two spikes* are seen on the ECG. The first

spike will be followed by a(n) _____ wave and the second spike will   *P*

be followed by a(n) _____ complex. Because the impulse produc-   *QRS*
ing ventricular depolarization is originating in the ventricles, the
QRS will be *(wide/narrow)*.   *wide*
In this mode of pacing two *foci*, the _____ and the _____,   *atrium   ventricle*
are paced in *sequence*. Because of these characteristics, this pacemaker is described as being both *bifocal* and *sequential*.

69 There is a fixed interval between the P wave spike and the QRS
spike. This is representative of the *P-R interval*. The duration of
the P-R interval is preselected by the physician.

70 The sequential pacemaker also has a *sensing mechanism*. Sensing
is accomplished via the electrodes in the *ventricles*. The pacemaker

is therefore "sensitive" to the patient's own _____ complexes.   *QRS*
If the patient has his own QRS complex, the pacemaker is programmed to *inhibit* both the *atrial* and *ventricular* spikes. Thus an-

other name for this type of pacemaker is the QRS-_____,   *inhibited*

_____, and _____ pacemaker.   *atrial   ventricular*

71 Another feature of this pacemaker is that it fires only when the patient's own rate falls *below a preset limit*. This pacemaker, then,

fires only when needed, or on _____.   *demand*
The most complete name for this pacemaker is the sequential bi-

focal _____ pacemaker.   *demand*
The advantage of this mode of pacing is that the atria and ventri-

211

cles are paced in *sequence.* Thus the atrial contribution to cardiac output *(is/is not)* lost as with other modes of pacing.   *is not*

72 *Let us review:* The sequential pacemaker *(may/may not)* be used in the management of A-V block.   *may*

The sequential pacemaker is QRS-*(inhibited/triggered).* If the patient has his own QRS, the atrial and ventricular spikes *(will/will not)* be seen.   *inhibited*   *will not*

The unique feature of the sequential pacemaker is that it has two

locations for its _____ electrodes.   *stimulating*

By pacing the atria and ventricles in _____, the _____ contribution to cardiac output is not lost.   *sequence*   *atrial*

73 IN SUMMARY:

A

CLASSIFICATION	COMPLEX FOLLOWING SPIKES	LOCATION	MODE OF ACTION	INDICATIONS
SEQUENTIAL BIFOCAL DEMAND	1. P WAVE 2. QRS COMPLEX	2 SITES: ATRIA VENTRICLES	INHIBITED	1. SINUS BRADYCARDIA 2. ACUTE OR CHRONIC A-V BLOCK

Fig. 9-11

B

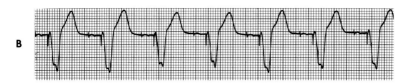

74 Let us briefly correlate the direction of stimulation and sensing in each pacemaker and the resulting ECG pattern.

PACEMAKER	DIRECTION OF STIMULATION AND SENSING	ECG PATTERNS
KEY	➤ =STIMULATION ┅➤ =SENSING A=ATRIA V=VENTRICLES P=PACEMAKER	
CONTINUOUS ATRIAL PACEMAKER	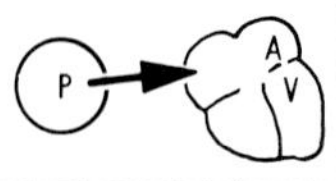	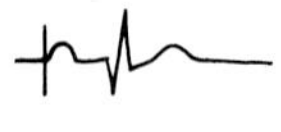
CONTINUOUS VENTRICULAR PACEMAKER	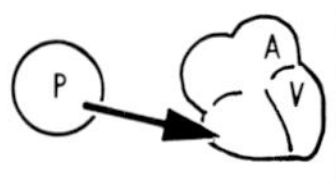	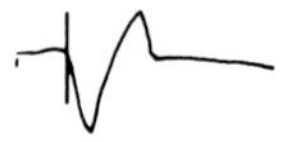
QRS- INHIBITED VENTRICULAR PACEMAKER	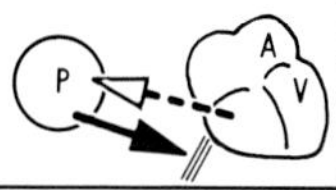	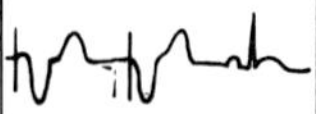
QRS-TRIGGERED VENTRICULAR PACEMAKER	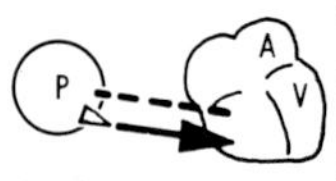	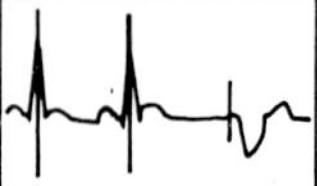

Fig. 9-12

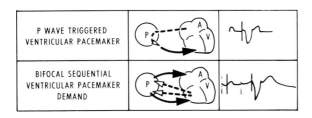

| P WAVE TRIGGERED VENTRICULAR PACEMAKER | | |
| BIFOCAL SEQUENTIAL VENTRICULAR PACEMAKER DEMAND | | |

Fig. 9-12, cont'd

Pacemaker malfunction

75 The purpose of a pacemaker is to provide an *electrical* stimulus that will result in a myocardial response when the heart's own *(electrical/mechanical)* system is failing. Just as the heart's own electrical system can fail, the artificial electrical system of the pacemaker unit can also fail to function normally. Before a problem-solving approach toward pacemaker failure can be developed, the nurse must first understand the mechanisms that allow for a pacemaker to function normally.

electrical

76 *Remember:* The type of pacemaker used most frequently in the setting of acute MI is the *(temporary/permanent)* pacemaker. The mode most frequently used is the QRS-inhibited (demand) pacemaker.

temporary

Let us review the components utilized in most *temporary* pacing units:

1. pulse generator
2. catheter containing stimulating and/or sensing electrodes
3. bridging cable (optional)

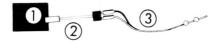

Fig. 9-13

1. Pulse generator
2. Bridging table
3. Catheter

77 The *pulse generator* contains the stimulating circuitry and the sensing circuitry, both of which draw energy from the battery pack.

The stimulating circuit transmits energy from the battery pack to the myocardium.

The sensing mechanism interprets the information about the patient's _____ rhythm.

natural

78 The *pacemaker catheter* transmits the electrical stimulus from the battery pack to the myocardium and transmits information about the patient's natural rhythm to the pulse generator. The catheter thus serves as a messenger between the pulse generator and the myocardium.

79 A *bridging cable* may provide an extension between the catheter and pulse generator to allow for patient comfort. If a bridging cable is utilized, the cable must be securely connected to the pulse

generator and _____.

catheter

80 For the pacemaker to stimulate and sense properly there can be no

breaks within or disconnections between the pacing components, i.e., pulse generator, bridging cable, and _____.

catheter

81 Another prerequisite for effective sensing and stimulation is that the catheter be properly positioned in the correct chamber and in contact with the endocardium.

82 The ventricular catheter is positioned ideally at the *apex* of the *right ventricle*. In this location the catheter is most stable and therefore remains in best contact with the _____.

endocardium

When the catheter is properly positioned in the _____ of the right ventricle, pacing should produce a positive complex in Lead I and a negative complex in Leads II and aVF (abnormal left axis deviation; see Unit 6). The QRS complex in Lead V_1 should also be negative.

apex

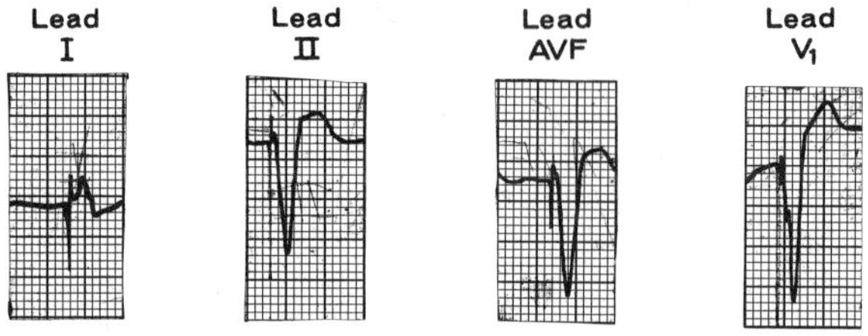

Fig. 9-14

83 *Let us review:* The components of a temporary pacing unit are:

1. _____ _____

pulse generator

2. _____

catheter

3. _____ _____
The pulse generator contains the _____ circuitry, the

bridging cable
stimulating

_____ circuitry, and the _____ _____.

sensing; battery pack

The battery pack generates the electrical _____ and pro-

stimulus

vides current for the operation of the _____ mechanism.
The sensing mechanism interprets information about the patient's

sensing

_____ _____.
For proper stimulating and sensing to occur, the catheter must:

natural rhythm

(1) be in contact with the _____ and (2) be located

endocardium

at the apex of the _____ _____.
The nurse can check for right apical pacing by checking Leads V_1,

right ventricle

____, ____, and ____.
Secure connections between the connecting cable, the _____

I   II   aVF
pulse

_____, and the _____ are necessary for normal transmission of the stimulus and for normal sensing.

generator   catheter

84 If all mechanisms of the pacing unit are functioning normally: (1) the pacing stimulus will be released as prescribed; (2) each pacemaker stimulus will result in a myocardial response; and (3) information about the patient's natural rhythm will be sensed and interpreted correctly.

85 The problems that occur as a result of pacemaker malfunction may be classified as follows:
1. problems related to stimulus release
2. problems related to stimulation or capture
3. problems related to sensing

Problems related to stimulus release

86 *Let us review:* The energy source or battery pack generates the

electrical energy that produces the electrical _____.   *stimulus*
The rate of stimulus release is adjusted to the individual need and is selected by means of a dial on the pulse generator.
The release of the stimulus appears on the ECG as a(n) _____   *pacing*

_____.   *spike*

The interval between two consecutive pacing spikes is known as the

_____ _____.   *automatic interval*

87 This interval should approximately correspond to the rate at which

the pacemaker is automatically _____.   *firing*
The automatic interval is therefore measured to confirm that stimuli are being released as prescribed.
Some variation in the automatic interval can be expected with normal pacemaker function. Marked variation in the automatic interval indicates malfunction.

88 Most problems with stimulus release are the result of *battery fail-*

ure or disconnections within or between the catheter and _____   *pulse*

_____. Occasionally, problems with stimulus release can be   *generator*
related to sensing malfunction.

89 Let us now consider the ECG manifestations of improper stimulus release.

90 Problems with stimulus release may be manifested by the intermittent or complete absence of a pacing spike.

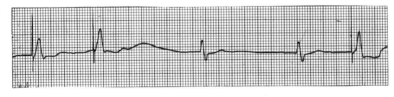

Fig. 9-15

91 Another manifestation of improper stimulus release is gross variation in the automatic interval.

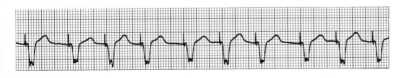

Fig. 9-16

92 When marked acceleration of the stimulus rate occurs, the pacing unit is referred to as a *runaway pacemaker*.
Appropriate intervention in the management of this problem is to disconnect the pacing unit to terminate the arrhythmia.

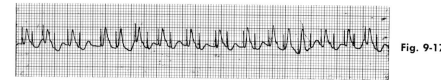
Fig. 9-17

Note: This arrhythmia is usually a manifestation of battery failure in an implanted pacemaker.

93 *Nursing orders:* Problems with stimulus release
1. Evaluate the battery pack and replace if necessary.
2. Check the integrity of the catheter and connections between the catheter and pulse generator.
3. Evaluate adequacy of patient's own rhythm; is the patient symptomatic?
4. Have Isuprel drip on standby.
5. Consider the functioning of the sensing mechanism.

Problems related to stimulation-capture

94 When a pacemaker is stimulating adequately, each pacing spike

should produce a(n) _____ response. When each pacing   *myocardial*
spike produces a myocardial response the pacer is said to be *in capture.*

If the stimulating electrodes are in the atria, each spike should

produce a(n) _____ _____. If the stimulating electrodes are in   *P wave*

the ventricles, each spike should produce a(n) _____ _____.   *QRS complex*

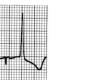 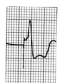
Fig. 9-18

When a pacing spike fails to produce a myocardial response, the

pacemaker is said to be out of _____.   *capture*

95 When an atrial pacemaker is *out of capture,* the pacing spike will

fail to produce a(n) _____ _____.   *P wave*
When a ventricular pacemaker is *out of capture,* the pacing spike

will fail to produce a(n) _____ _____.   *QRS complex*
Therefore, improper stimulation will result in failure to _____.   *capture*

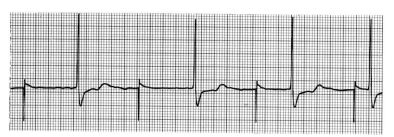
Fig. 9-19

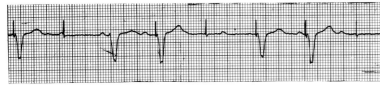

Fig. 9-19, cont'd

96 When a pacemaker loses capture, a problem-solving approach that
considers each component of the pacemaker unit should be used.
Failure to capture may be a result of *inadequate voltage* being re-

leased from the _____ _____.   *battery pack*

97 The *pacemaker catheter* must also be considered. A break within the

catheter may lead to loss of _____. A frequent cause of fail-   *capture*
ure to capture is a floating or improperly positioned catheter.
Remember: Proper capture requires that the catheter be in contact

with the _____ and located at the apex of the _____   *endocardium   right*

_____.   *ventricle*

98 The *bridging cable* must also be considered as a potential source of

trouble. A faulty connection between the bridging _____, the bat-   *cable*

tery _____, and the _____ may result in failure to   *pack   catheter*

_____.   *capture*

99 *Nursing orders:* Failure to capture
1. Evaluate the pulse generator.
   — increase amplitude or voltage being delivered from the

   _____ _____   *battery pack*
2. Evaluate the catheter.
   — check to see if the catheter is pacing at apex of right

   _____   *ventricle*
   — check Leads V_1, I, II, and aVF; monitor on Lead aVF
   Note: Catheter position can be evaluated only if there is at least intermittent capture.
   — reposition the patient
   — if arm is site of catheter insertion, reposition the patient's

   _____   *arm*
3. Evaluate adequacy of underlying rhythm; is patient symptomatic?
   — obtain order for standby atropine or Isuprel
   — if patient loses consciousness, start cardiopulmonary resusci-
     tation
4. If these measures fail to regain pacemaker capture, the physician should be notified.

Problems related to sensing

100 *Let us review:* The sensing mechanism is contained within the

   _____ _____ and draws energy from the battery pack.   *pulse generator*
   The purpose of a *sensing mechanism* is to interpret information
   about the patient's own *rhythm*. The sensing mechanism allows
   the pacemaker to fire *(with/without)* regard for the patient's own   *with*

_____. The patient's own rhythm is then *protected* from com-

rhythm

petition by the _____.

pacemaker

101 Most problems with sensing occur because of failure of the sensing mechanism within the pulse generator or improper positioning
of the catheter.

102 When the sensing mechanism fails, the pacemaker will fire *(with/
without)* regard for the patient's own rhythm. The pacemaker then
competes with the patient for control of the rhythm. This manifestation of failure to sense is known as *competition*.

without

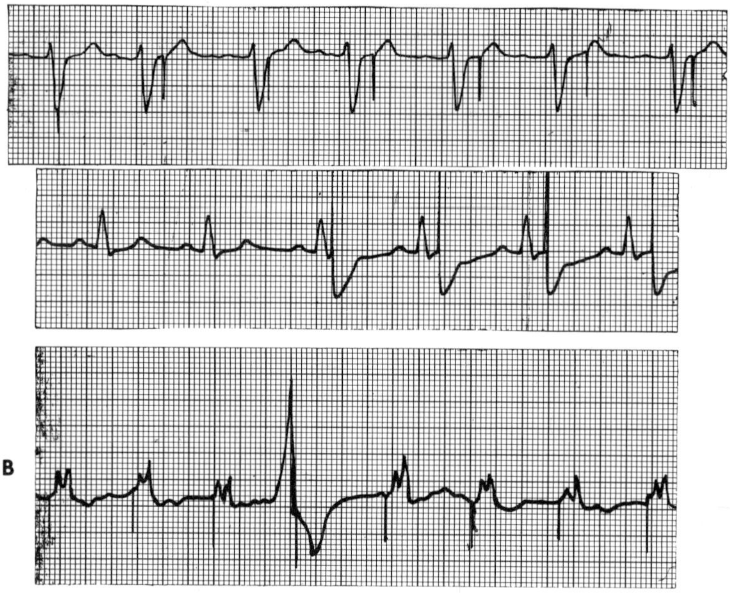

Fig. 9-20

Note: Failure of the sensing mechanism may also be manifested
by failure to sense an *occasional* impulse. (See Fig. 9-20, *B*.)
The danger of this disregard for the patient's own rhythm is that
a pacing spike may fall during the vulnerable period of the car-

diac cycle, causing _____ _____ or ventricular

repetitive firing

_____.

fibrillation

103 *Let us review:* Failure to sense may result in a complication known

as _____. The danger associated with this complication

competition

is that a pacing spike may fall during the _____ period,

vulnerable

resulting in _____ _____.

*ventricular fibrillation/
repetitive firing*

Failure of the pacemaker to sense may be a result of malposition

of the _____ or failure in the sensing _____.

catheter; mechanism

104 *Nursing orders:* Failure to sense (competition)
   1. Evaluate the pulse generator.
      — increase the sensitivity
   2. Consider catheter position.
      — attempt to reposition the catheter by moving the patient or
        his arm if necessary

— check for catheter placement; Leads V_1, II, and aVF should be negative during pacing; Lead I should be positive

3. If the sensing problem cannot be corrected, the pacemaker should be gradually turned off. The pulse generator should be replaced before pacing is continued.

4. If the patient's own rhythm is not adequate:
   — increase pacer rate to overdrive
   — if the impulse not sensed is ventricular in origin, lidocaine may be administered

5. Unipolarize a bipolar pacing setup.

6. Notify physician.

7. Check intracavitary signal.

Suggested readings

Barold, S.: Modern concepts of cardiac pacing, Heart Lung 2:(2)238, Mar.-Apr. 1973.

Berkovits, B. V.: Bifocal demand pacing, Presented at The Soma Weiss Memorial Symposium at Peter Bent Brigham Hospital, Boston, April 23, 1970.

Castellanos, A., and Lemberg, L.: Electrophysiology of pacing and cardioversion, New York, 1969, Appleton-Century-Crofts.

Castellanos, A., and others: Pacing in acute myocardial infarction; a programmed introduction, Chest 58:152-163, 1970.

Castellanos, A., and others: Post-infarction conduction disturbances; a self-teaching program, Dis. Chest 56:421, 1969.

Castellanos, A., and others: Ventricular-triggered pacemaker arrhythmias, Brit. Heart J. 31:546, 1969.

Castellanos, A., and others: Pacemaker-induced cardiac rhythm disturbances, Ann. N. Y. Acad. Sci. 167:903, 1969.

Castellanos, A., and others: Evaluation of countershock treatment of atrial flutter, Arch. Intern. Med. 115:426-433, 1964.

Castellanos, A., and others: Implantable demand pacemaker, Brit. Heart J. 30:29, 1968.

Castellanos, A., and others: Cardioversion of A-V nodal tachycardias, Am. J. Cardiol. 18:884, 1966.

Castellanos, A., Spence, M., and Chapell, D.: Management of ventricular standstill, Rocom Monitor, Nutley, N. J., June, 1970.

Castellanos, A., and Lemberg, L.: Pacemaker arrhythmias and electrocardiographic recognition of pacemakers, Circulation 1352-1391, June, 1973.

Castillo, C. A., and others: Bifocal demand pacing, Chest 59:360-364, 1971.

Castillo, C. A., Castellanos, A., and Berkovits, B. V.: Use of electrical pacemakers in the management of cardiac arrhythmias, Geriatrics 25:117-131, 1970.

D. C. Countershock, Am. Heart J. 70:583, 1965.

Driefus, L. S., and others: The advantages of demand over fixed-rate pacing, Dis. Chest 54:86, 1968.

Friedberg, C. K., Cohen, H., and Donoso, E.: Advanced heart block as a complication of acute MI; role of pacemaker therapy, Prog. Cradiov. Dis. 10:466, 1968.

Kastor, J. A., and Leinbach, R. C.: Pacemakers and their arrhythmias, Prog. Cardiov. Dis. 13:240, 1970.

Kimball, J. T., and Killip, T.: Aggressive treatment of arrhythmias in acute MI; procedures and results, Prog. Cardiov. Dis. 6:483, 1968.

Lemberg, L., and Castellanos, A.: An artificial pacemaker responds to the electrical needs of the heart, Medical Times, Nov., 1965.

Lemberg, L., and Castellanos, A.: Cardioversion; a study of 203 episodes, J. Fla. Med. Assoc. 52:21-24, 1965.

Lemberg, L., and others: The treatment of arrhythmias following acute myocardial infarction, Med. Clin. N. Amer. 55:273, 1971.

Parsonnet, V., and others: Implantable cardiac pacemakers status report and resource guideline, Circulation 50:21-35, Oct. 1974.

Preston, T. A., and Yates, J. D.: Management of stimulation and sensing problems in temporary cardiac pacing, Heart Lung 2(4):533, July-Aug. 1973.

Rios, J. C., and Hurwitz, L. E.: A simplified logical approach to the evaluation of temporary pacemaker malfunction, Heart Lung 3(4):624, July-Aug. 1974.

Vassoun, C., and Lown, B.: Cardioversion of supraventricular tachycardias, Circulation 39:791-801, 1969.

Vinsant, M. D., and others: Pacemakers in 72, Heart Lung 1:362-373, May-June 1972.

Wagner, G. S., and McIntosh, H. D.: The use of drugs in achieving successful DC cardioversion. In Friedberg, C. K., editor: Current status of drugs in cardiovascular disease, New York, 1969, Grune & Stratton, Inc.

Fusion, aberration, and atrioventricular dissociation

FUSION BEATS

1 Depolarization of the same chamber of the heart by two or more simultaneous impulses may result in a *fusing* of these impulses, or

a(n) _____ beat.   *fusion*

2 When a ventricular focus discharges an impulse just as a supraventricular impulse reaches the ventricles, a *fusion beat* will occur. The ventricles will be partially depolarized by the supraventricular impulse and partially depolarized by the *late* _____ impulse.   *ventricular*

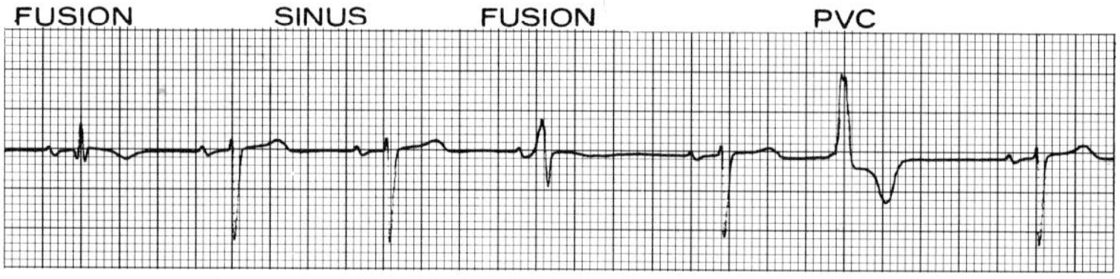

Fig. 10-1

The resulting QRS complex will appear as a *blend,* or *fusion,* of the two contributing impulses in contour and duration.

3 A diagnosis of fusion beats can be made only when there is electrocardiographic *evidence* that at least two distinct foci are attempting to control the ventricles. This establishes the *probability* that fusion beats could occur.
A prerequisite to the diagnosis of fusion beats is establishing the

_____ that fusion could occur. Therefore, the first step in   *probability*
the identification of fusion beats is to identify each distinct focus
in its naturally occurring form. *Then* look for beats that are a *blend*

of these in _____ and _____.   *contour*   *duration*

4 Fusion beats occur when two or more impulses _____ in _____   *blend*   *contour*

and _____.   *duration*
Therefore, when fusion beats occur, there *(will/will not)* be a   *will*
change in the QRS configuration.
The QRS complex of a fusion beat is partially formed by the patient's supraventricular impulse. Therefore, the QRS complex of a
fusion beat may be partially *(narrow/wide).*   *narrow*
However, the fusion complex will appear *(the same as/different*   *different from*
from) the normal QRS complex of the supraventricular impulse.
This is because of the presence of a concurrent *(ventricular/supra-*   *ventricular*
ventricular) impulse.

5 The clinical significance of a fusion beat is that there is a ventricular focus attempting to control the ventricles.

Therefore, fusion beats are significant not for their supraventricular component but for their _____ component.

ventricular

6 Common examples of fusion beats are:
1. Sinus beat with a late PVC

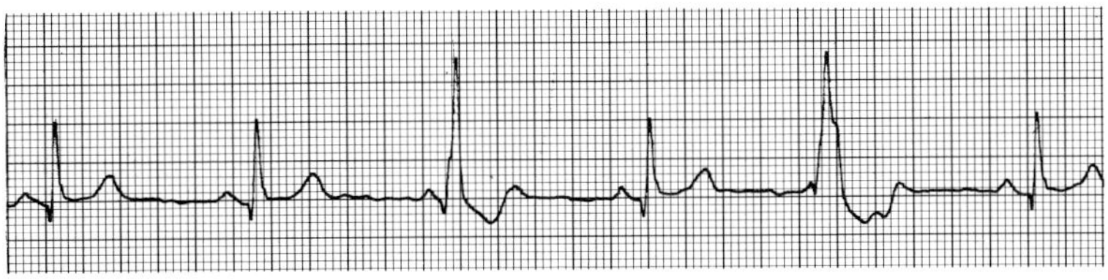

Fig. 10-2

2. Sinus beat with a pacemaker beat

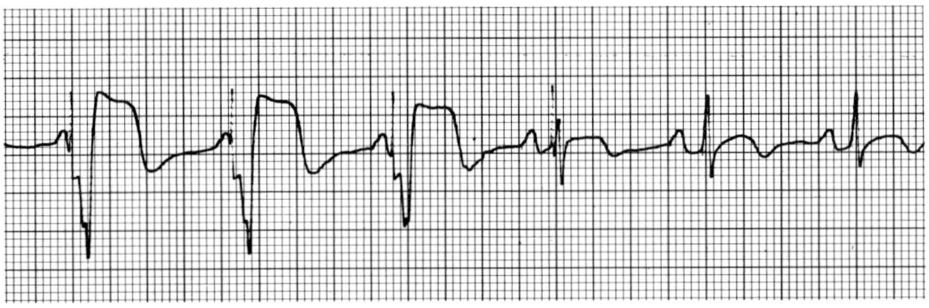

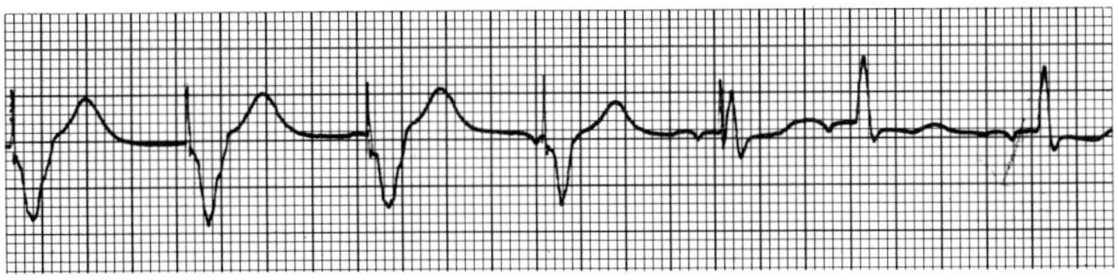

Fig. 10-3

Note: Fusion beats may also occur less commonly when two ventricular ectopic impulses fuse and appear as a third focus.

Remember: Fusion beats are not significant for their _____ component but for their _____ component.

supraventricular

ventricular

7 The purpose of a pacemaker is to induce a ventricular focus. Therefore, fusion beats are expected in the presence of normal pacemaker function and *(are/are not)* clinically significant.

are not

When fusion beats result from spontaneous ectopic ventricular impulses, however, they *may* be clinically significant. A sequence of three or more consecutive fusion beats indicates the presence of a nonparoxysmal _____ tachycardia. Consecutive fusion beats, therefore, *(may/may not)* be clinically significant.

ventricular
may

Fusion beats may also be benign. For this reason, some physicians choose to medicate fusion beats *only* if they occur consecutively and if the patient is symptomatic.

8 When fusion beats occur in the setting of a bradyarrhythmia, therapy is directed toward accelerating the supraventricular impulse. This mode of therapy is used to *overdrive* the ventricular impulse. This may be accomplished by pharmacological or electrical intervention.

When fusion beats occur in the presence of an adequate supraven-

221

tricular rate, therapy is directed toward depressing ectopic activity in the ventricles.

9 *Let us review:* Fusion beats are usually regarded clinically as *(ventricular/supraventricular)* and are produced by *(early/late)* ventricular beats.

ventricular

late

Most commonly, they result from the _____ of a _____ and _____ impulse in the _____. The resulting QRS complex appears as a _____ of these two impulses in _____ and _____.

fusion; supraventricular

ventricular; ventricles

blend   contour

duration

10 *Nursing orders:*
   1. When identifying fusion beats, look for a P wave and a short P-R interval preceding the fusion complex. This finding is evidence of a supraventricular component.
   2. Report fusion beats:
      — when they are isolated but occur more frequently than 5 per minute
      — when they are consecutive; this may indicate the presence of nonparoxysmal ventricular tachycardia
      — when they are associated with a bradyarrhythmia
   3. If fusion beats are occurring consecutively in the presence of an adequate supraventricular rate, have Xylocaine at the bedside.
   4. When fusion beats occur in the presence of a bradyarrhythmia, have *atropine* at the bedside.
   Remember: Fusion beats that occur in the presence of normal pacemaker function are benign.

ABERRATION

11 Unlike fusion beats, aberrant beats appear to be *ventricular* but are actually *supraventricular*. Unlike fusion beats, aberrant beats are *(early/late)* ectopic beats.

early

An aberrant beat is an *early,* or premature, supraventricular impulse that is blocked in one bundle branch.
Therefore, an aberrantly conducted beat represents a functional

_____ _____ block.

bundle branch

12 If an *early* supraventricular impulse reaches the ventricles and the right and left branches are *not* refractory, the impulse *(will/will not)* be conducted normally—for example, a *normally conducted* PAC.

will

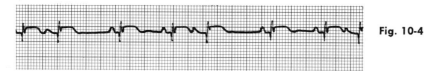

Fig. 10-4

13 If an early supraventricular impulse reaches the ventricles when *both* the right and left branches are in their refractory period, the impulse *(will/will not)* be conducted—for example, a *nonconducted* PAC (Fig. 10-5).

will not

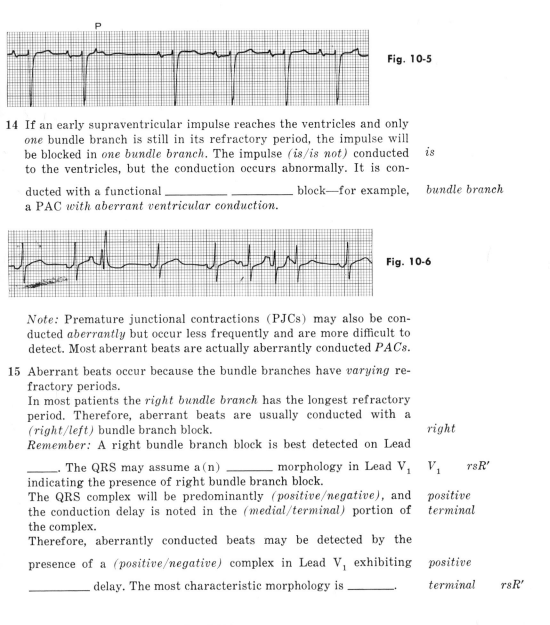

P

Fig. 10-5

14 If an early supraventricular impulse reaches the ventricles and only *one* bundle branch is still in its refractory period, the impulse will be blocked in *one bundle branch*. The impulse *(is/is not)* conducted to the ventricles, but the conduction occurs abnormally. It is con-

        is

ducted with a functional _____ _____ block—for example, a PAC *with aberrant ventricular conduction.*

        bundle branch

Fig. 10-6

Note: Premature junctional contractions (PJCs) may also be conducted *aberrantly* but occur less frequently and are more difficult to detect. Most aberrant beats are actually aberrantly conducted *PACs.*

15 Aberrant beats occur because the bundle branches have *varying* refractory periods.

In most patients the *right bundle branch* has the longest refractory period. Therefore, aberrant beats are usually conducted with a *(right/left)* bundle branch block.

        right

Remember: A right bundle branch block is best detected on Lead

_____. The QRS may assume a(n) _____ morphology in Lead V_1 indicating the presence of right bundle branch block.

        V_1 *rsR′*

The QRS complex will be predominantly *(positive/negative)*, and the conduction delay is noted in the *(medial/terminal)* portion of the complex.

        positive
        terminal

Therefore, aberrantly conducted beats may be detected by the

presence of a *(positive/negative)* complex in Lead V_1 exhibiting

        positive

_____ delay. The most characteristic morphology is _____.

        terminal   *rsR′*

Lead V_1

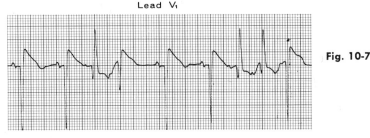

Fig. 10-7

16 The right bundle branch block pattern seen in aberrantly conducted beats may also be detected only by the presence of the terminal de-

lay if seen clearly in Leads I and _____.

        V_6

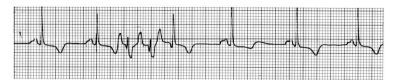

Fig. 10-8

The initial deflection in right bundle branch block (septal depolarization) is usually *(the same as/different from)* the patient's normal beat. Therefore, the initial deflection of an aberrantly conducted beat is often *(the same as/different from)* the patient's normal beat.

the same as

the same as

17 Aberrant beats may also occur in the presence of *atrial fibrillation.* In the presence of atrial fibrillation, the R-R cycles vary. The length of the refractory periods also varies.

A long R-R cycle *(prolongs/shortens)* the length of the refractory period of the next R-R cycle.

prolongs

When a long R-R cycle is followed by a short cycle in the presence of atrial fibrillation, the impulse ending the short cycle *(is/is not)* likely to be conducted aberrantly.

is

Lead V₁

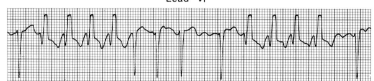

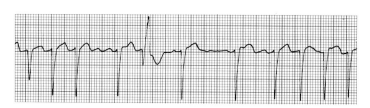

Fig. 10-9

18 Aberrant conduction may also occur in the presence of rapid, sustained supraventricular tachycardias. Runs of supraventricular tachycardia with aberration may appear as *ventricular tachycardia.*

19 *Let us review:* Aberrantly conducted beats occur *(early/late)* and appear to be *(ventricular/supraventricular).* In reality, however, aberrant beats occur when a *(ventricular/supraventricular)* impulse is functionally blocked in one of the bundle branches. The most common type of aberrantly conducted impulse is a *(PAC/PJC).* Therefore, most aberrantly conducted beats should be *preceded* by an

early
ventricular
supraventricular

PAC

early _____ wave.

P

Aberrant beats are usually conducted with a *(right/left)* bundle branch block pattern. Therefore, they may be detected by the presence of a *(positive/negative)* complex in Lead V₁ exhibiting

right

positive

_____ delay.

terminal

Aberrant beats commonly occur in the presence of _____ fibrillation. This is because in atrial fibrillation *short* R-R cycles are

atrial

often preceded by _____ R-R cycles.

long

Nursing orders: Aberration
1. When analyzing *premature beats* that have a wide and/or different QRS morphology:
    — look for preceding P waves
    — if no P waves are *clearly* visible, consider the premature beats as *PVCs* when clinically evaluating the patient
    — for a more thorough analysis:
        — monitor the patient on Lead V_1
        — look for an rsR′ configuration in the premature beats or an upright pattern with terminal delay
Note: The presence of an rsR′ configuration does not necessarily confirm the presence of aberration.
2. Rule out aberration:
    — if the premature impulses are end-diastolic
    — if the premature impulses are preceded by a short rather than a long R-R cycle
3. Consider the clinical setting in which the abnormal beats occur.
    — is the patient in atrial fibrillation?
    — has the patient been having PACs?
4. In the presence of atrial fibrillation, monitor on Lead V_1.
5. In the presence of tachyarrhythmia with wide QRS complexes:
    — evaluate how the patient is tolerating the arrhythmia—is he symptomatic?
Note: In the presence of ventricular tachycardia, the patient will be more symptomatic than in supraventricular tachycardia.
    — try to obtain a recording of the onset of the tachyarrhythmia
    — if the patient loses consciousness, always treat the arrhythmia as *ventricular.*

A-V DISSOCIATION

20 In various cardiac arrhythmias the *atria* beat independently of the *ventricles.*
Examples of such arrhythmias include:
1. ventricular tachycardia without retrograde conduction
2. junctional tachycardia without retrograde conduction
3. complete heart block (CHB)
The term *A-V dissociation* is therefore a general term and might apply to any of an entire group of arrhythmias with varying clinical significance.

21 *A-V dissociation* is a general term that may be used to describe *any*

cardiac arrhythmia in which the _____ and the _____   *atria*   *ventricles*
beat independently.
The best indication of a constant relationship or association be-

tween the atria and the ventricles is the presence of a fixed _____   *P-R*
interval. Therefore, in the presence of A-V *dissociation* the P-R interval *(does/does not)* remain the same.   *does not*

22 A-V dissociation is a *(specific/general)* term. It is a description, *not*   *general*
a diagnosis. If the term *A-V dissociation* is to be used to describe an arrhythmia, a more complete interpretation is required:
    — A-V dissociation resulting from *ventricular tachycardia*
    — A-V dissociation resulting from *junctional rhythm,* or *tachycardia*
    — A-V dissociation resulting from *complete heart block*

23 When A-V dissociation occurs as a result of ventricular tachycardia, the ventricles generally beat *(faster/slower)* than the atria.   *faster*

VENTRICULAR TACHYCARDIA

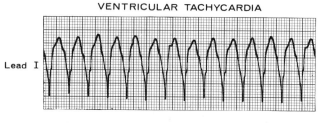

Lead I

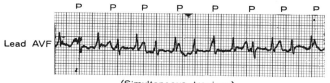

Lead AVF

Fig. 10-10

(Simultaneous tracings)
Note: the dissociation between the P waves
and QRS complexes in Lead AVF

24 Let us now consider another example of A-V dissociation:

When the sinus node slows, the _____ _____ tissue may   *A-V junctional*
assume control of the ventricles. If this occurs and the atria *remain*
under the control of the *sinus node*, the atria and the ventricles will
become *(associated/dissociated)*.   *dissociated*

25 This rhythm is best identified as A-V dissociation with a(n) _____   *A-V*

_____ pacemaker.   *junctional*
When this arrhythmia occurs, the ventricular rate is usually only
slightly greater than the atrial rate. Thus the P waves appear to
march into the QRS complex, forming a characteristic pattern.

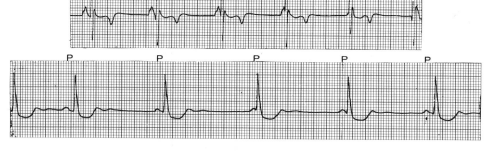

Fig. 10-11

Note: When the atrial rate and ventricular rate remain almost the
same, this arrhythmia may be referred to as *isorhythmic* A-V dissociation.

26 A-V dissociation with a junctional pacemaker has the same clinical

significance as a(n) _____ rhythm.   *junctional*
This arrhythmia is terminated when the sinus node accelerates and
again controls the heart.
If therapy is indicated in the management of this arrhythmia, the

drug of choice would be _____.   *atropine*

27 When A-V dissociation occurs as a result of complete heart block, the ventricles beat *(faster/slower)* than the atria.   *slower*

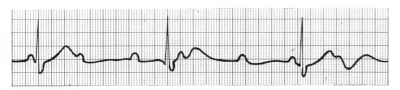

Fig. 10-12

Suggested readings

Cohn, L. J., Donoso, E., and Friedberg, C. K.: Ventricular tachycardia, Prog. Cardiov. Dis. 9: 29, 1966.

Damato, A. N., and Lau, S. H.: Clinical value of the electrogram of the conduction system, Prog. Cardiov. Dis. 13:119, 1970.

Fisch, C.: Self assessment—aberrant conduction, Heart Lung 2(2):260, Mar.-Apr. 1973.

Gozensky, C., and Thorne, D.: Rabbit ears: An aid in distinguishing ventricular ectopy from aberration, Heart Lung 3(4):634, July-Aug. 1974.

Hurst, W. J., and Logue, R. B., editors: The heart arteries and veins, New York, 1970, McGraw-Hill Book Co.

Kisten, A. D.: Problems in the differentiation of ventricular arrhythmias from supraventricular arrhythmias with abnormal QRS, Prog. Cardiov. Dis. 9:1, 1966.

Marriott H. J. L.: Practical electrocardiography, Baltimore, 1968, The Williams & Wilkins Co.

Marriott, H. J. L., and Sander, I. A.: Criteria, old and new, for differentiating between ectopic ventricular beats and aberrant ventricular conduction in the presence of atrial fibrillation, Prog. Cardiov. Dis. 9:18, 1966.

Marriott, H. J. L.: Differential diagnosis of supraventricular and ventricular tachycardia, Geriatrics, Nov. 1970.

Schamroth, L.: An introduction to electrocardiography, Edinburgh, 1971, Blackwell Scientific Publications.

Scherf, D.: Remarks on the nomenclature of cardiac arrhythmias, Prog. Cardiov. Dis. 13:1, 1970.

Singer, D. H., and Geneick, R. E.: Electrophysiologic aspects of aberrancy, Am. J. Cardiol. Vol. 28, Oct. 1971.

Abbreviations

ADH	antidiuretic hormone	LAEDP	left atrial end diastolic pressure
ALAD	abnormal left axis deviation	LAH	left anterior hemiblock
ALMI	anterior/lateral myocardial infarction	LBB	left bundle branch
		LBBB	left bundle branch block
A-V	atrioventricular; arteriovenous	LDH	lactic dehydrogenase
aVF	augmented voltage foot lead (of ECG)	LPH	left posterior hemiblock
		LV	left ventricle
aVL	augmented voltage left lead (of ECG)	LVEDP	left ventricular end diastolic pressure
aVR	augmented voltage right lead (of ECG)	MI	myocardial infarction
		MVO_2	myocardial oxygen demand
AWMI	anterior wall myocardial infarction	NA	normal axis
BP	blood pressure	PA	pulmonary artery
CHB	complete heart block	PAC	premature atrial contraction
CHF	congestive heart failure	PAEDP	pulmonary artery end diastolic pressure
CLBBB	complete left bundle branch block		
CNS	central nervous system	PAT	paroxysmal atrial tachycardia
CO	cardiac output	PCWP	pulmonary capillary wedge pressure
CPK	creatinine phosphokinase		
CPR	cardiopulmonary resuscitation	PJC	premature junctional contraction
CVP	central venous pressure	PVC	premature ventricular contraction
ECF	extracellular fluid	RA	right atrium; right arm
ECG	electrocardiogram	RAD	right axis deviation
HBD	alpha-hydroxybutyrate dehydrogenase	RBB	right bundle branch
		RBBB	right bundle branch block
IAD	indeterminant axis deviation	RV	right ventricle
ICF	intracellular fluid	S_1, S_2 etc.	heart sounds
ISF	interstitial fluid	S-A	sinoatrial
IV	intravenous	SGOT	serum glutamic oxalacetic transaminase
IVC	inferior vena cava		
IVF	intravascular fluid	SVC	superior vena cava
IWMI	inferior wall myocardial infarction	VF	ventricular fibrillation
JG	juxtaglomerular apparatus (of kidney)	VR	ventricular rate
		VSD	ventricular septal defect
LA	left atrium; left arm	VT	ventricular tachycardia
LAD	left axis deviation		